Two of a Kind

The Story of How My Little Boy and I Survived Cancer

Geri Payawal Shepard

DEDICATION

This book is dedicated to Brad, my strong and loyal husband, to Maddox, my brave and exuberant Maddy-moo, and to Danika, my smart and sassy Danzi-roo.

You are and always will be the three greatest loves of my life.

CONTENTS

Introduction

October 17, 2012

It was a year ago today that I discovered a lump in my left breast. It was soon after that day that I would be diagnosed with breast cancer. It is on this day, exactly one year after making that life-changing discovery, that I begin this project.

My journey through breast cancer treatment was made more meaningful because as I was getting chemo, so was my five year old little boy. My son, Maddox, was diagnosed with Acute Lymphoblastic Leukemia on June 17, 2009. I was diagnosed with Breast Cancer on October 25, 2011. We both finished our treatments in 2012!

Going into this, I knew that writing my story would not be easy. It would force me to relive a lot of the fear and sadness I went through after being diagnosed with breast cancer. As difficult as I knew telling my story would be, I knew for a sure fact that writing my son's story would absolutely break my heart. There are countless memories that I placed so carefully in the deepest parts of my mind, always knowing they were there, but always making sure that I pushed them way back, whenever some of those painful thoughts made their way to the front. As much as our family found ourselves in some pretty dark places during that time, not all of the memories were bad. There were many moments of just incredible love, hope and yes, pure joy. I know that to tell our story with truth and care, I must and would have to reach for those memories, both the good and the bad, and allow them and all the emotions that come with them, to resurface. This is going to be an emotional roller coaster. I'm scared to go back there, but I do it with a clear purpose. It is my hope that sharing my son's story and my story will inspire others to believe in the strength of the human spirit and the power of family.

This is the story of our journey and what it took for us to survive it.

Chapter One

Maddox's Journey

In June of 2009, my son, Maddox, was diagnosed with ALL, Acute Lymphoblastic Leukemia.

This is his story.

When I look back, I believe that Maddox's illness first presented itself in March of 2009. Our family was on, what I think was our first family vacation, in Orlando. Maddox was only two years old at the time. I remember him getting a fever during that trip. Aside from the fever, he was fine, with no other symptoms. The next day, there was no more fever so of course we didn't think anything of it. Little did we know that something was brewing inside him. That something would soon change all of our lives.

Shortly after that trip, particularly around April and May of 2009, we noticed Maddy getting more of these random fevers. He would always recover, but only to get another fever within a couple of weeks, always with no defining symptoms - no cough, no cold, no runny nose. It was all very peculiar, but not so much to cause us concern or raise any flags. By the time he a got his third fever with no other symptoms, it was time to investigate. We went to our pediatrician to get him examined. She told us that it was not uncommon for toddlers to catch a virus and then get over it - they go on play dates, go to the playground - so we were told that this was perfectly normal. We didn't have a reason to think otherwise because Maddy always seemed to bounce back.

When Maddy got another fever shortly after that visit, I remember saying to my husband one night before bed, that I was getting worried about our son, and that this just didn't seem right. Somewhere inside, my maternal instincts were telling me that this was not normal. Maddox also seemed less energetic, started to appear pale, and was also bruising in parts of his body that didn't make any sense, like his back and his inner thighs. At the time we attributed all of those symptoms to Maddy just fighting off the fevers and the bruises to him just being an active toddler. We decided, as most parents do, to trust what our pediatrician told us. It seemed logical for us to believe that when most toddlers catch something, they get over it. Even then, I had a nagging feeling, but foolishly let myself brush it off.

There was one particular incident that scared me to the very core. I was sitting in the dining room, with Maddox and my daughter, Danika, in their high chairs. I can't remember whether I was feeding them breakfast or lunch. All I remember was that Maddox could barely keep his eyes open. It was more than just him feeling sleepy. I kept yelling his name saying, "Maddy, Maddy, wake up, wake up!" He just kept slumping over, closing his eyes. When he wasn't hearing me, my alarms went off and in my panic, I even slapped his cheek several times - not too hard, but enough to try to get him to respond. It was like he just kept fainting. He would open his eyes, but have this look of just extreme tiredness. I was petrified. My fear was building, and fast. I quickly called my husband, Brad, who is often my voice of reason, and told him that Maddox was acting very strange to say the least, that he had no energy, and that he kept falling asleep at the table. In hindsight, this should have been a HUGE red flag, but what parent in the world would have thought the unimaginable. After hanging up with my husband, I immediately called the pediatrician who told us to bring Maddox in. I got the kids ready and rushed Maddox to the pediatrician's office. By that point, he had perked up a bit. I explained his symptoms to the nurse practitioner. She examined him, looked at his fingernails to determine whether he was dehydrated, which he wasn't, and eventually instructed us to take him to the ER for further examination.

I practically ran the stroller to the ER. The initial examination didn't indicate anything in particular. In my effort to try to figure out what was going on, I explained to the physician that my daughter, Danika, previously had a stomach bug. When I said that, it was like a light bulb went on in his head and based on the symptoms that I explained, and what I just told him, the doctor concluded that Maddox probably caught the stomach bug from his sister. He attributed the lack of energy with Maddox having nausea and gave him some Zofran. He said Maddy should perk up after getting the Zofran and sent us on our way. I strolled the kids back home, exhausted from the dramatic events of the day, but relieved that we had gotten to the bottom of this - or so I thought. They never did a blood test.

To this very day, I blame myself and agonize over and over again on whether or not I should have said anything about the stomach bug. I kept thinking that if I hadn't given the doctor a reason to think it could be anything else, then he probably would have ran a blood test. It tortures me to think that had I not said anything, then maybe the doctor could have detected Maddy's illness sooner. Stupid, stupid me. I should have insisted on a blood test, but what did I know? As much as I blame myself, I also hold the pediatrician's office accountable for not doing a blood test. At that point we had already expressed our concerns with them on several occasions regarding Maddox's fevers. Each time, we were sent on our way believing that our son was perfectly fine. They should have performed a blood test as part of his exam, maybe not after the first fever, but surely after the third or fourth one, and most certainly after this most recent incident. I guess I could play the blame game all day, but it will not change the course of events that were to follow.

Chapter Two

In mid June, we went on a long weekend vacation to visit the kids' grandparents, Dave and Cathie in Rochester. It was during that visit that it was quite apparent to Maddy's grandma in particular, that his coloring did not look right. During this visit, Maddy was extremely tired all the time and just wanted to lay down - not normal behavior for any active two and a half year old! I remember coming back to the house after Brad and I had done some shopping, and noticed Maddy standing up, but with his upper body and head sort of leaning or laying on the couch. Maddox had been having some constipation so I thought perhaps that was the reason for his demeanor. Maddy also did not have much of an appetite. At the time, we didn't think anything of it as he tends to be a picky eater. Man, as I'm writing all of this, I feel like there were so many warning signs, but there always seemed to be a logical reason to explain Maddy's behavior. Were we in denial? Were we being horribly clueless parents? Why would we think anything else was going on when all the doctors kept telling us that Maddox was okay? All we could do was trust the professionals.

It was a couple of days into the visit, when Maddy developed yet another fever, that we discussed our growing concerns with the grandparents. That was probably the turning point for us. It was then that Maddy's grandma, Cathie confided in us that as soon as she saw Maddox get out of the car when we first arrived, she immediately noticed a drastic paleness in his appearance. When she said that, it really made us notice the changes in Maddy that hadn't jumped out at us as much before, as the changes had occurred slowly over time. I guess we had become so accustomed to them and hadn't noticed the drastic differences.

Right then, we knew that this was something more, and yes, we were worried, but in no way could we have guessed the unthinkable or even imagined Maddy's condition. Not long after this, we realized what a miracle it was that we discussed our concerns with Dave and Cathie. It was that conversation that fueled our determination to get some answers. This time, we would not be so easily sent away.

Chapter Three

Monday, June 15, 2009

I remember taking the six hour drive back home from Rochester to New York City and calling our pediatrician to insist on another exam, and more specifically, a blood test. We arrived back to NYC late afternoon and went immediately to the doctor's office, who then gave us the rushed prescription for blood work. As I looked at the doctor, I thought, "Where was this sense of urgency when we were there all the other times???" The pediatrician agreed that Maddy was very pale and did not look well. Since the laboratories were already closed, the soonest we could do the blood test was the next morning.

I took Maddox to the laboratory Tuesday morning for the rushed blood test. Tuesday afternoon we were in the ER. By Tuesday night we were admitted to the hospital. Yes, it all really happened that fast. One minute we were being overcautious parents and the next minute our son was in isolation at the hospital.

This was how that unforgettable day played out. I remember getting the call from the pediatrician that afternoon with the results of Maddy's blood work and her telling me that Maddy's counts were extremely low, and that he was anemic. She said it was an emergency and instructed me to take Maddox to the ER immediately. Oh my God!!! I started to freak out and my heart was racing. She wouldn't tell me anything more, which made me even more anxious and afraid. I called Brad and told him what I knew and to rush home. I called my friend, Jennifer and told her that it was an emergency. I asked if she could come and watch Danika so that Brad and I could take Maddox to the ER. She was the one person I knew that I could count on and trust to be there. I will always be so grateful to Jennifer for coming at a moment's notice, no questions asked, which was good because we had no idea what the hell was going on. Brad got home very quickly. Danika was still napping when Jennifer and her two young boys, Joe and Hank, arrived. I hoped that Danika wouldn't be scared to wake up and not find Mommy, Daddy, or Maddy there. Thankfully, Danika knew Joe and Hank well and later that day, Jennifer told me that Danika was happy to see Hank when she woke up. As Brad and I left with Maddy, I could tell that Jennifer noticed the concern on our faces. We knew this couldn't be good.

Chapter Four

We quickly got Maddox to Mount Sinai Hospital. At the ER, all we knew was that Maddy was extremely anemic and that his blood counts were very low. They placed us in a room while various nurses and doctors checked in on us. They weren't telling us much of anything, which made us even more worried. Hours passed and we still didn't know anything. We did our best to amuse Maddy, but he was getting restless and cranky. There wasn't very much for Brad and me to do to calm our nerves either. By early evening, one of the doctors came in and told us that they were going to admit Maddy to the hospital. He explained that Maddy was going to be seen by an oncologist. Silence. Disbelief. Shock. I swear I don't think I heard anything else he said after that. It was when this word, oncologist, started getting tossed around that Brad and I felt the wind knocked right out of us. In that incredible moment, our world was turned upside down. None of this made any sense. I struggled to hold back the tears. I wanted to get out of there. We didn't know anything specific yet, but it was enough to shock our system with fear. We wanted to believe that everything was going to be okay, but we had a sinking feeling that it wasn't. I have absolutely no idea how we functioned after that. All I remember was making a call to Jennifer to check on Danika, and to tell her what was going on. I could barely manage to get out any words over my sobbing at the mention of the oncologist. Brad called his parents doing his best to contain his emotions. Brad's mom, Cathie, immediately booked a flight to be with us. As we waited for a hospital bed to be prepared for Maddox, I was able to line up our regular babysitter, Julia, to take over for Jennifer as I knew that Jennifer had to take her boys home. The hospital bed was ready by around 11PM. I would stay with Maddox at the hospital while Brad went home to relieve the babysitter. It was important for one of us to be there with Danika. I didn't want him to leave. We desperately needed each other for support, but we had to be there for both of our kids.

It was close to midnight by the time Maddy and I were escorted to the hospital room. Before Maddox could even get settled in bed, he had to get a chest x-ray. It was very late and we were both exhausted. I remember this particular incident so vividly because I hate myself for what I didn't do. Anytime I think about this, my blood boils with anger. The technician assigned to do Maddox x-ray was horribly inconsiderate and rude. I remember he kept saying to one of his colleagues that he "should be going home by now." He had no consideration that I could totally hear him. Well excuse me asshole, but that was your fucking job! He made it obvious that it was late and that he wanted to get the x-ray done very quickly. Maddy was just a little boy. He was tired and scared. Maddy didn't know what was going on and so of course when the technician goes to take his chest x-ray, he doesn't lay still. The technician expressed frustration and showed no patience or any compassion. I wanted to scream at him to show some care and yell that Maddox was just a baby and that he's scared. Why oh why didn't I do that?!!!! Why didn't I stand up for my little boy like any good mother would have done?!!! Even today, I get so angry at myself that I did not say anything to that horrible man. I should have defended my son, but all I wanted was for it to be over so that Maddy can finally be left alone to get some rest.

Instead of confronting the technician, I just held Maddy down to stay still so that this insensitive man could get the x-ray done. Maddy was crying and inside I was breaking down. I am so sorry Maddy. Mommy is so sorry to have let that happen. I am deeply ashamed that I let the technician get away with that behavior. I am not a confrontational person, but in that moment I should have put him in his place. I should have told him to have some decency and to show some compassion. I should have told him that he will stay there as long as it takes for him to get the x-ray done without frightening my son. Hell, I should have called him a fucking asshole to his face! Fucking asshole!!! Every time I replay this memory in my head, my heart hurts and I beat myself up all over again. It pains me so much to think about that night because I was too embarrassed to speak up. I know my husband would not have tolerated that. Brad would have said something. I hate myself for not being assertive enough to speak my mind. I was literally shaking by the time the technician left.

After I calmed Maddy down and told him that he can go to bed, I went to the nurse's station and reported the technician to one of the nurses. I specifically said that he treated us terribly, and that he should not be in that profession dealing with kids. I went on to say that the patients in that wing are children, many of whom are scared and they, above all people, should be treated with the utmost sensitivity and care. Damn it! Why didn't I say all of this to that man?! If I did, then maybe he would not treat another child like that. Even though I did voice a complaint, I know I will never ever forgive myself for not reprimanding that man directly for his appalling behavior. This incident taught me a huge lesson about ALWAYS putting decorum aside when it comes to looking out for my children's well being. Screw politeness! I vowed from then on out to always have my kids' backs!

Chapter Five

When I got back to our hospital room, Maddy was asleep. Thank goodness. I laid down on the chair pull-out bed feeling drained from top to bottom. My body was aching, but not as much as my heart. In the dark with just the lights from the hall flickering, I cried. There would be no rest for me that night.

It was around 2AM when I heard a light tap on the door. As it opened, someone called out, "Mrs. Shepard." A bit startled, I sat up and said "Yes." I saw this very tall, imposing man come in and sit himself down on a chair across from me. I don't recall all of the exact details of our conversation, but this is what I do remember.

We didn't turn on the lights so as not to disturb Maddox. In the dim room, it was quiet except for our hushed voices. He introduced himself as Dr. Del Toro. He was all business and my immediate impression was that I did not like him. I wanted him to be this warm and fuzzy kind of doctor that holds your hand, but he wasn't. He felt very distant. Little did I know at the time, that this same doctor, would soon become my family's champion. Dr. Del Toro would very quickly earn our utmost respect and trust. However for the moment, he was just another doctor.

In that first meeting, he showed very little bedside manner or emotion as he asked me what I knew so far. I told him that I didn't know much and basically repeated everything we had been telling the other doctors all day in the ER. I told him about Maddy's random fevers, his lethargy and paleness, the bruises on his body, and his low blood counts. Dr. Del Toro was very quiet, emotionless as I continued on like a speech I had said so many times already. I was so scared. All I wanted was some shred of reassurance from him that everything was going to be fine. I was desperate for any comforting words, but Dr. Del Toro did not sugar coat anything. After I spoke, he simply and matter-of-factly stated that he believed that Maddox may have leukemia. What? My heart stopped, then it began to race. That can't be it. I must have heard him wrong. I tried to keep calm as he discussed other possibilities of what else "it" might be. I was in denial. I thought for sure there was no way that it could be leukemia. That was just impossible, even ridiculous. It had to have been one of the "other" possibilities that Dr. Del Toro talked about. I convinced myself that that's what it was. It had to be something else, something harmless. I even went so far as to try to convince the doctor of that as well. I felt like I was grasping at straws. Even though I heard Dr Del Toro say it was very likely leukemia, I remember I just kept saying to him, "But it could be that other thing you mentioned, right? *Right?*" He replied that it was possible, but he doubted it. Finally he said that we will know for sure once Maddox gets a bone marrow biopsy. The biopsy was scheduled for later that morning. We would have answers once those results came in.

As Dr. Del Toro left the room, I have never felt so alone. All by myself, I heard the doctor tell me that my little boy may have leukemia. I resisted every urge to panic, even though I was filled with indescribable fear. I was desperate to call Brad, but I wanted him to get some rest, and I thought there was no sense in alarming him too. After all, I didn't know anything for certain yet. So I sat there with the enormous weight of that information on me. I was so scared and didn't have anyone to comfort me. I had all of these thoughts running through my head and no one I could talk to sitting there in the dark at 2:30 in the morning. For dear life, I clung, just clung to the thought that there was no way that this could be cancer. I held on strongly to the hope that it must be, had to be one of the "other possibilities." I talked myself through it and eventually, I actually felt some confidence, not 100% confidence, but enough to get me through that morning to believe that it was all going to be okay. I couldn't, I WOULDN'T believe that my little boy had cancer. No way.

Chapter Six

Brad arrived early the next morning with Danika and his mom, Cathie. She had arrived from Rochester sometime that morning. Although they knew that Maddox was going to get a bone marrow biopsy that morning, I don't remember telling either of them all the details about the conversation I had with Dr. Del Toro in the middle of the night. I know that I must have, at some point, told them, especially Brad, what Dr. Del Toro suspected, but for some reason, I can't seem to remember this conversation. Perhaps this was just one of the memories I blocked out from my head. I do remember a phone call that I made to my sister telling her we were in the hospital. Even now, I could hear my unsteady voice as I told her that the doctor said that Maddox might have leukemia. She was incredulous. She said very sure of herself, "No, it is not that." She even managed to partly convince me that the notion of it was preposterous. I explained how Dr. Del Toro said it could be some other thing and we agreed that that seemed more like it, and that every thing was going to be fine.

Chapter Seven

Wednesday, June 17, 2009

Maddox got the bone marrow biopsy that morning. Afterwards, the mood in Maddy's hospital room was quite calm and I would say, even playful. Maddox and Danika played and watched cartoons. Despite the circumstances, it almost felt just like an ordinary day. Maybe it's because we actually did convince ourselves that whatever Maddy had, it was just some harmless thing that kids get and it would all be okay. This moment was, as they say, the calm before the storm.

It was getting close to dinner time and since I had just spent the night with Maddy at the hospital, it would be my turn to go home and get some rest, while Brad stayed with Maddy. We were all smiles as I got ready to head home with Danika and Cathie. I remember standing by the elevator when one of the nurses catches up to us and tells me that Dr. Del Toro wanted me to stay. I thought nothing of it. Perhaps Dr. Del Toro was going to tell us that we could bring Maddy home today. I put Cathie and Danika in a cab and headed back to Maddy's hospital room. When I passed the nurse's station, I saw Maddy's pediatrician talking to Dr. Del Toro and still, I didn't think there was anything unusual going on. That should have been a clue that something was up when I saw our pediatrician there. I had no idea that my heart was about to ripped out of my chest.

I went in the room and told Brad that Dr. Del Toro wanted me to come back, and that his mom and Danika went home. A few minutes later, Dr Del Toro accompanied by Maddox's pediatrician came into the room. Brad and I smiled at them and said our hellos very casually, truly not expecting anything major. We thought they were just coming in to check on us. Honest to God, we were not prepared for what was about to happen.

Maddy's pediatrician quietly sat on a chair on the other side of the room. Brad was lying on the bed with his arm around Maddox and I was sitting in a chair next to Brad. This is how we got the news.

Dr. Del Toro sits on the chair across from me, looks at us, and simply says, "Mr. and Mrs. Shepard, Maddox has leukemia." For those few seconds Brad and I must have stopped breathing. The room was silent, everything was still for just a second and then I heard a sound that I didn't recognize. It was the sound of my husband falling apart. It snapped me out of my shock. I didn't cry. I just looked at Dr. Del Toro. I saw his eyes with a hint of redness as it began to well up with tears at the sound of Brad's crying. It was the first time I had seen any emotion from Dr. Del Toro. As soon as I saw his eyes, I knew it was true. I covered my face with both hands and whispered, "Oh my God," and then I too broke down. We didn't even have a chance to brace ourselves. It all happened in a flash. We knew that Dr. Del Toro told us that this was likely, but we honestly thought it had to be something else. In an instant, Brad and I were leveled. I saw my strong husband with his head down hugging Maddox so fiercely while we both cried a deep and heavy cry. We couldn't stop. We could barely catch our breath. Finally, I asked Dr. Del Toro and our pediatrician to give us some privacy. As they left the room, with tears burning and streaming uncontrollably down my face, I climbed on the bed and held my innocent baby boy. Together, Brad and I clung to our son and each other as if all of our lives depended on it.

Maddy was only two years old at the time. I didn't want to ever let go. I remember Maddox start to whimper. He looked at us scared, knowing that his mommy and daddy were crying, but not understanding why. All we wanted to do was protect him and make this all go away. I remember I kept saying, "I'm so sorry Maddy. I'm so sorry. Mommy didn't know you were sick. I didn't know. I didn't know. I'm so sorry. I love you so much. Please forgive me, Maddy. Please forgive me." In anguish, I just kept repeating this. I had yelled at Maddy a few days earlier and thought he was just being lazy and acting out, when in reality his body was already fighting cancer. He was acting tired and not himself because of this horrible disease, not because he was misbehaving. I should have shown him more patience. I should have been a better mommy. I am so ashamed at how I treated him. I will never ever forgive myself for that. Brad and I held on to our son as tight as we could hold him as if to somehow shield him from any harm. We stayed like that for a very long time.

Chapter Eight

During the course of that evening, we were given more information about Maddox's condition. He was diagnosed with Acute Lymphoblastic Leukemia. The treatment for boys is about three and half years. Three and a half years. Dear Lord, this would be our life for the next three and a half years. We barely had time to recover from the news of Maddy's diagnosis, and now we had to somehow come to terms with how long this road would be. For the second time, Brad and I felt the wind knocked right out of us. Dr. Del Toro told us that Maddy's age was in his favor and that kids are very resilient. He said that the success rate for treating this kind of leukemia is very good. That knowledge would be the driving force that would get us through this.

Chapter Nine

I don't know how, but somehow, Brad and I got ourselves together as best as we could. It was time to tell the family. The first call was to Brad's mom who was home with Danika. Brad held the phone and he never even got the words out before he lost it. I remember having to take the phone from him so that I could tell Cathie what we had just learned. I cried the whole time as she just kept saying, "We're going to fight this, Geri. We're going to fight this." Cathie would later tell me that earlier that day, when we were by the elevators getting ready to leave, she saw Dr. Del Toro tell the nurse to get me and she knew by the look on his face that something was wrong. I was oblivious of the whole thing.

The next call I made was to my sister. Her first response was, "Oh my God." She said that she would pray for Maddox and then she just kept telling me to be strong. "Be strong." How in the hell were we going to do that when Brad and I couldn't even stop crying? We must have cried every single day for weeks following Maddox's diagnosis.

At some point, Maddox's pediatrician came to check on us. She told us that Brad and I could look into other treatment centers, but she felt very strongly that Maddox would get excellent care at Mount Sinai. To be honest, I don't think the thought of researching other facilities even crossed our minds. Perhaps it would have been the wise thing to do, but everything was happening so fast, and all we wanted was to get the care that Maddy needed as soon as possible. We never even questioned transferring him, and the thought of Maddox having to endure more exams by another doctor was out of the question. He and *we* had been through enough. We were confident in our decision to keep him where he was and we trusted Dr. Del Toro. That was all there was to it.

While the pediatrician was there, I also remember her giving me two notebooks. She said I could use one of them as a journal to write down everything I was feeling. I don't think I ever wrote a single word in that journal. At the time, I was too distraught to think about putting anything on paper. The other notebook on the other hand, became like my bible. It was in that notebook that I would track every chemo, every medicine, every fever, every hospital stay, and every clinic appointment. Basically it became the notebook for all things related to Maddox's treatment. Logging all of those details became my priority for the next three and a half years. That big, thick notebook would become a testament to everything we as a family experienced during Maddy's treatment.

After getting Maddox's diagnosis, the hospital made an exception and allowed both Brad and me to stay the night with Maddy. This was good because there was no way either of us was going to leave, no fucking way. That night as we watched our son sleeping, Brad and I held each other and cried. Still reeling from the news and what lay ahead of us, Brad and I couldn't make sense of anything. We knew we had to be strong, but we weren't going to start that night. We were too overwhelmed and emotionally drained. I had never seen my husband look so defeated and there was absolutely nothing I could do to make it better.

Maddox's chemo treatment would begin immediately that week. We watched in agony as our son cried while getting examined, x-rayed, poked, and prodded. He was scared. We were terrified. There was one particular incident that I know Brad and I will never forget. The nurses were trying to draw Maddy's blood so they kept sticking him with the needle. He screamed and flailed around in pain and fear every time they tried to get to his vein. It got to the point where Brad had to restrain him. I watched my husband holding my son down as he cried, "All done! All done!" over and over again. It broke my heart to a million pieces. I watched the nurses moving the needle all around while it was still inside his arm trying to find that vein. I wanted to make them stop, but we didn't have a choice. We knew it had to be done. Maddy must have been wondering why the two people that are supposed to protect him were letting this happen. It was torture. No parent should have to endure that, and no child should ever have to suffer that horror. This is probably one of the worst memories I have of those early days in the hospital. No matter how hard you try to forget, some memories just stay with you.

We couldn't believe this was happening to us. We struggled to maintain a sense of "everything is going to be okay," all the while our world was crashing down.

Chapter Ten

Maddox was soon placed in a private room in protective isolation. Since the chemo would suppress his immune system, it was important to keep Maddox in as sterile and clean environment as possible.

On Thursday of that week, Maddy received surgery to place a mediport in his chest so that the chemo could be administered with ease. This was a godsend as the physical and emotional pain of sticking our son with needles all over his body was definitely taking a toll on him, and on us. This port was a device that was placed under the skin of his upper right chest. It would be the device where Maddox would be accessed to draw his blood and where his chemo and other medicines would be administered. Once emla, a numbing lotion, was applied to the area, the port would allow getting accessed to be done with very little discomfort.

In the midst of all the heartache of having to go through all of this, as hard as it is to believe, I do remember moments of humor. I remember Maddox getting some medicine right before the surgery to get the port placed. It was supposed to knock him out. We observed this medicine take effect on Maddox making him very loopy and happy. He had this goofy smile on his face. Brad and I sat outside the procedure room watching our little boy walk around tipsy, looking and acting like a drunk sailor. It was really quite amusing and for those few minutes before the surgery, we actually laughed and smiled. Before the medicine knocked him out completely, the surgeon came and picked him up to get him ready for the surgery. Dr. Del Toro told us it was a fairly simple procedure and that he would be in the operating room as well. We gave Maddy a hug and kiss and told him that we loved him as we watched him get carried off into the OR, still with that goofy look on his face. Brad and I sat in the waiting room, holding hands, doing our best to keep it together. This was just the beginning. I prayed and prayed for God to watch over my baby boy. I don't remember how long we were there. I just remember Dr. Del Toro coming out to tell us that all went well and that we can bring Maddox back to his room when he woke up in recovery. Once Maddox was settled back in his room, I prepared to head home to get some rest, while Brad stayed with Maddy. It was Thursday. I hadn't been home since Tuesday morning. As much as I hated to leave, I knew it was just as important for Danika to have one of her parents with her. When I arrived, with tears in her eyes, Cathie greeted me with a huge hug. I did not get three steps in before I collapsed in her arms. This was the first time I had seen Cathie since Maddy was diagnosed. Once again, she just kept saying that we would fight this. I don't remember much else about that night. I do remember that it was the night that I shared the news in an e-mail to all of our family and friends.

On Thursday, June 18, 2009, with a heavy heart and tears running down my face, I wrote:

Hello Everyone,

We wanted to share some news with all of you. Yesterday evening we found out that our son, Maddox, has Acute Lymphoblastic Leukemia. In an instant our lives are changed. We are emotionally battered, but are staying strong. Maddox has been through so much already with his medical treatment and is SO brave. He will be getting chemo treatment. The doctors say that he has the most common form of leukemia in young children and the success rate is very good. We ask that you please keep him in your thoughts and prayers. We are taking it day by day and it is the support of our family and friends that keep us going and keep us strong.

Love,
Brad, Geri, Maddox and Danika

The heartfelt responses were immediate. The message reached all of our family and friends who rallied around us with the force and might of an army. I was moved to tears with each and every response. It was this outpouring of love that would lift us up and keep us strong and steady as we prepared for this battle. The prayers and words of encouragement kept coming and each single one gave us the courage to fight.

The next morning, Cathie, Danika, and I went to the hospital together. I brought a change of clothes and toiletries as it would be my turn to spend the night with Maddox. This would be the routine that Brad and I established - we would be there together during the day and then each of us would take turns spending the night at the hospital with Maddy. Brad coordinated time off from his job and Cathie made plans to stay and help us. We were so thankful to have her. We knew that Danika would be in good, loving, and safe hands with Grandma while Mommy and Daddy took care of her big brother. We got everything in place so that we could focus on our son.

Chapter Eleven

The days at the hospital all sort of blended into the next. I may not go into the specific dates, but what I will write about are the events and moments that I do remember, and some that I for sure won't ever forget.

One day, it must have been the first or second week at the hospital, Dr. Del Toro took Brad and me to the outpatient pediatric oncology clinic. This clinic was located in the Division of Pediatric Hematology and Oncology at Mount Sinai. This is where we would bring Maddy for his chemo once he was done at the hospital. The clinic had a little play area with various toys and games, as well as a little play kitchen, and tables and chairs for arts and crafts. All of these activities were available for the kids while they were there for treatment. We also met some of the nurses assigned to that department. Looking around, I realized that this would be our lives for the next three and half years. I couldn't even imagine it, but there we were being introduced to this world of childhood cancer. This became even more real after what happened next.

Dr. Del Toro finished showing us around and then took us into a room to show us a slide of Maddox's blood. I didn't really know what to expect. The images from the slides were projected on to a TV monitor. First, he showed us what a normal slide looked like. Then he placed Maddox's slide in the microscope. What I saw on the screen took my breath away. I fought back tears. There right in front of me was Maddox's cancer. A normal slide shows the cells in a variation of different colors. In Maddox's slide, the cells were one dominant color, with just a small scattering of other colors. Looking at it, I was horrified and terrified at the same time. In that moment, it wasn't just this sort of abstract diagnosis anymore. Here was evidence of the disease. There was the cancer invading my son's body. That was the leukemia. I wept for my sweet innocent baby boy whose precious little body was fighting this monster. To see it was staggering beyond belief. I desperately wanted to give his body all the strength it needed to fight this thing. When we left the room, I took a deep breath. Sobered by what we had just looked at, we felt the gravity of the situation reach a higher level. As traumatizing as it was to see it, it was important for us to know what we were dealing with. To this day, those images have yet to fade from my memory.

Chapter Twelve

Brad and I got lots of information regarding the options we had for Maddox's treatment. The Oncology Group at Mount Sinai had a treatment protocol that was in the research phase. We had the opportunity to participate in the research study or choose to go with the standard treatment for ALL. What they would do is randomly determine whether we had that option. Should the random selection choose the standard treatment, we would have to do the standard treatment and would not have the option to choose the research study. Should we be selected to participate in the research study, we would have to decide whether to go with the research or stay with the standard treatment.

The information we had to read in order to make this decision was extremely daunting. We had to read through various chemo drugs and their side effects, some of which I had to block out because it scared me so much. There were so many different kinds of drugs and medicines. I was so petrified of what these drugs could do to my son that I could barely bring myself to read through all of the material. It was like choosing the lesser of two evils. We had to evaluate which protocol we felt was the safest and which we felt was going to be the most effective. Our son's safety and precious life were in our hands. We felt the tremendous weight of this awesome responsibility. So many thoughts went through our heads - should we do the research study with the hopes that there will be an incredible breakthrough that would cure our son or should we stick with the standard protocol that has been tried and tested to work? We second guessed ourselves numerous times when we discussed both options. Brad and I were incredibly overwhelmed with this decision. At a time when our biggest decision should have been choosing which preschool Maddy should attend, we were faced with the horrific task of choosing which chemo treatment he should get. It was awful and all too surreal.

Eventually, Brad and I decided that we felt the most "comfortable," as much as we could be under the circumstances, with choosing the standard protocol. We just didn't want to take any chances with a research study and felt that the standard treatment was the safest choice for us. We were prepared to have this answer should we be given the option. When the time came to inform Dr. Del Toro of our decision, we sat in his office and anxiously awaited to hear where we were placed. After all of our struggles to make the decision, to our relief, it turns out that Maddox was placed in the standard protocol. That was that.

Chapter Thirteen

After we discussed all the details regarding Maddox's treatment plan, Dr. Del Toro also got very personal with Brad and me. He informed us that the road ahead would not be easy and that many couples break up due to the stress and emotional turmoil the situation brings. I couldn't believe that it could happen to us. I remember that Dr. Del Toro never actually said the word "divorce," but what he did do was gesture with the pointy finger of each hand. He had them side by side together and then he said, "A lot of couples...." and then moved the pointy fingers slowly away from each other, separating them until both hands were apart. We got the gist of it. At the time, I knew that Brad and I felt confident in our love for each other and more than secure in our marriage, that we as a couple, could weather this storm. This would not be an issue for us. Brad and I were solid. As I write this today, I have to say, and I know that Brad would agree, that after everything we've been through, our vows have definitely been tested. I will talk more about this later, but for now all I will say is that we are thankful that our marriage has survived, but not without taking some hits.

Chapter Fourteen

Maddox's treatment involved several phases which included the Induction Phase, the Intense Phase, and the Maintenance Phase. The Induction Phase is just what it sounds like - it would be the phase when Maddy's body would be introduced to the chemo. The day that Maddox got his first infusion, I remember saying a prayer over and over again, as I watched this drug travel through the tube of his IV up into his body. In my mind, I just kept saying, "Let this chemo kill the cancer, but please God, please oh please protect his body. Please keep Maddox safe."

Once Maddox's chemo began, he was monitored very closely. Every three to four hours, they would take his blood pressure and temperature. They were constantly drawing his blood. He had to get x-rays, ultrasounds, and tests. They got him started on countless supportive drugs and medications that were given in conjunction with the chemo. Maddox was so young, just a baby. He had no idea what was going on and was often scared to be touched and examined so much. In order to make him feel safe and to take some of the fear away, we changed the names of many things and made them more "child-friendly" so to speak. We called getting his blood pressure, "arm hugs." We called his IV a "necklace." We used words that he could relate to, words that were innocent to a child. We did our best to make his room as happy a place as we could. We hung pictures up on the wall right in front of his bed so that he could see them every day. They were pictures of our family, pictures of him and his friends playing, and pictures of him laughing and having lots of fun. These photos of the good times were just as much for us, as they were for Maddox. These pictures would ground us and bring us back to happier places. We also brought some of his favorite toys and stuffed animals to decorate his room. We did everything we could think of to shield our son from the reality of what was going on.

There was a program at the hospital called the Child Life Program where volunteers would come and bring various toys, coloring books, crayons, and DVD's to the children placed in isolation.

Because Maddox was immunocompromised, he couldn't go to the playroom that was down the hall. They wanted to protect him as much as possible from any outside germs. As you can imagine, we really appreciated the Child Life program. As part of the program, we could sign up to have musicians come and play their guitar for us. These musicians would come with an assortment of instruments that the kids can play along with them as they sang. Of course when they came, they were required to wear gloves and sometimes, masks. There was one woman that came and played for us quite frequently. Maddox enjoyed these visits and would joyfully play with the drums or the xylophone. For those moments, it was like he was a normal kid. For me these visits were often very emotional. She sang many songs while she visited with us, but the one song that always moved me to tears was, "You Are My Sunshine." The beautiful lyrics of this simple nursery song held so much more meaning for me. As a mother faced with this unbelievable situation, listening to the words tore at my heart every single time. As the musician sang out loud, inside, silently, I said the same profound lyrics with her, as I looked at my son with so much love in my heart, "You are my sunshine...You make me happy, when skies are grey. You'll never know dear, how much I love you. Please don't take my sunshine away." To this day, I can't listen to that song without crying. During those difficult times at the hospital, this innocent nursery song would become my deepest prayer, "Please God, please don't take my sunshine away."

Because Maddox was placed in protective isolation, we limited his visitors. The only visitors we allowed were family. Sometime that first week at the hospital, my aunt and her family came to visit us. There was a courtesy family room right outside of Maddy's room where they were waiting. Brad stayed with Maddox. I remember walking in the courtesy room and immediately breaking down as soon as I saw my Aunt Emma. She was my family. My mom and dad were in the Philippines. My aunt was the first family member on my side of the family that I saw since Maddox was diagnosed. Since my parents couldn't be there, my aunt was like a second mom to me. I let go. I cried and I cried while I clung on to her. Her husband and daughter just watched us like this for what seemed like a very long time. She did her best to comfort me and I did my best to let her. I finally was able to compose myself as I filled her in on Maddox's treatment. Soon after that, my sister arrived. She too was like a second mom to me. When I saw her walk in the room, I lost it once again. She just kept telling me not to cry. The intensity of the events of the past few days caught up with me, and it was all I could do. Until I saw them, I didn't realize just how much it meant to me to have my own family there. Eventually, Brad came in to join us. They told us to be strong and gave us many words of encouragement and love. Maddox was resting so we thought it best that they leave him be. As they prepared to leave, they said they would pray for Maddox and our family. It was an emotionally exhausting visit, but one that I really needed.

Looking back at some of those days is not easy. I never realized that a person could be capable of so many tears. It seemed like Brad and I were always crying. We cried in the hospital together, we cried on the walks home when one of us was going to take care of our daughter, while the other was with our son at the hospital, and we cried alone at night as the family was separated trying to make sure our whole family was taken care of.

Thinking of the simple walks to and from the hospital holds some sad memories as well. I remember several walks where I would have to put my sunglasses on so that I could hide my tear-stained face. It was summer and the days were bright and sunny. I would walk along Fifth Avenue and pass several playgrounds along the way and hear the laughter and play of so many children. It was such a stark contrast to what was happening in our lives. Those long summer days that should have been filled with days at the beach and frolicking in the park were instead days spent in isolation at the hospital. I was envious of all the families and children that I watched going about their day without a care in the world. I was sad for my son who was missing out on all those joys of being a kid playing with his friends at the playground. I was sad for my daughter who I couldn't take to the playground or simply spend as much time with because I was needed at the hospital. I was sad for Brad and me because instead of enjoying our children playing and having fun, we had to grapple with the fact that our son had cancer. Maddox was barely three years old and Danika was just one and half at the time. Those are such amazing ages when they are discovering things in the world and they are developing their personalities. I feel like we were all robbed of fully experiencing all those precious moments. They say when one member of the family goes through a medical crisis, the whole family goes through it. We all have certainly suffered in each of our own ways.

Chapter Fifteen

Brad and I got very little rest when it was his or my turn to spend the night at the hospital. It didn't help that those chair pull-out beds were not very comfortable. Because they took Maddox's vitals for what seemed like every four hours, we were often woken up several times in the middle of the night. Even today, whenever I hear the do-ba-do sound of a blood pressure machine, I am taken back to memories of those days of being at the hospital.

Maddox too was often woken up, very cranky and understandably so, while having his blood pressure and temperature taken. They did not use an ear thermometer to take his temperature, but instead used the one that you have to place under the arm. If he was lying in a certain position, getting his temperature taken without disturbing him sometimes took some effort. It always seemed like it took forever to get his vitals taken. It was very rare that Maddy was able to sleep through all of that. I often had to calm him down so that the nurse could get the vitals done as quickly as possible. In addition to having his vitals taken, Maddox had to get his blood drawn either in the middle of the night, or at the crack of dawn, or sometimes both. The nurse would come in the wee hours and set up all of her gear of needles, vials, syringes, and alcohol wipes. The good thing was, thanks to the mediport, they were able to just access Maddox through his IV. No more arm pinches, thank the Lord! Some nurses were awesome and very adept at doing this quickly and gently in the dark, with very little light in the room, while others let's just say, seemed to have less finesse. After a while, depending on which nurse was on duty, I knew what kind of night we were going to have.

We knew that we had been at the hospital for a long time when Maddy started calling his hospital room home and would weakly say "almost home" on our way back to his room after one of his numerous procedures. It was heartbreaking. I guess I could understand that because after a couple of weeks, we all settled into a "routine" at the hospital. We got to know our nurses, we familiarized ourselves with Maddy's medications, we learned how to navigate our way through the hospital to get to his various appointments and exams, and we knew where to get extra blankets and pajamas for Maddy when we needed them - basically, we made that hospital room home during our stay.

Believe it or not, Maddox even learned to potty train at the hospital. How crazy is that?! One day, Maddy just decided he didn't want to potty in his diaper any more. This was such an exciting achievement that we should have celebrated in our own home, but instead it happened in a hospital room. We didn't even have those cute little potty seat trainers. Because Maddy's IV sometimes didn't quite stretch all the way to the bathroom and because I didn't want to risk the IV getting disconnected, I remember Maddy potty training using those hospital bed pans. Yep, you heard it right, the bed pans. I don't know what I was thinking, but it worked. It was the closest thing that looked like it could be a potty trainer. We would put it on the floor and somehow Maddox managed to squat himself down on those things and do his business. Gradually and eventually, as Maddy realized it made much more sense to use an actual bathroom, we got comfortable navigating the IV and wheeling the machine it was attached to closer to the bathroom. Learning to potty train is one of the most momentous accomplishments in a child's development. We weren't completely out of diapers yet, but this was a huge step in that direction. For all parents, that is a big deal. My little boy was growing up. Despite where we were when it happened, I felt the glowing pride of any parent witnessing their child achieve this milestone for the first time.

As the days went by, we got to know a lot of the hospital nurses. Some of them were quite exceptional - not to be bias, but the Filipina nurses, Raj and Theresa were amazing. They were not just extremely capable and competent, they were also very caring, kind, and considerate. They were wonderful with Maddy. As a mother wanting the best care for her son, this made such a difference. I always felt a sense of relief and confidence when they were on duty. As they took such great care of Maddy, they became part of this journey with us.

We also got accustomed to the schedule of the doctors' daily rounds. On occasion and with our approval, Dr. Del Toro would bring a group of residents with him into the room. During these visits, Dr. Del Toro would have me describe how Maddox's illness presented itself. I would talk about the random fevers and the bruises on his body and the lack of energy. I was never able to get through one of these visits without tearing up. I even noticed several of the residents get teary too when listening to me describe the series of events that led us to this place. Even today telling our story without getting emotional is difficult, if not impossible. I remember Dr. Del Toro would then say to the residents, "See how difficult this is for the parents." It was to teach them to have compassion for what the families go through. I think that is one of the most significant and valuable lessons those residents would ever learn during their training. Compassion. It makes a hell of a difference.

When you are at the hospital for several weeks, a lot of the faces you see in the hallway get familiar, not just the nurses, doctors, and staff, but also the other patients and their families. At the hospital, the pediatric floor was divided into two wings. One wing was for the mild and moderate cases, and the other wing was for children being treated for life-threatening illnesses. Most of the children in this wing were placed in protective isolation.

There was this one woman whose son was in treatment. He was much older than Maddox, probably in his late teens. They often mentioned how age was in Maddy's favor because he was so young when he was diagnosed. Kids are very resilient at such a young age. From what I remember, this older boy had been in the hospital for several months and it seemed that he was having a difficult time of it. Every time I saw his mother, it looked like the weight of the world was on her shoulders. Every inch of her face was sad and dark. She looked beaten and weary. My heart felt for her and what she must have been going through. We never spoke and I never approached her. I guess I was too scared to know what her situation was, and I also wanted to shield myself from anyone else's pain. Mine was enough. Occasionally, the chaplain would make her rounds visiting the rooms. One day she was in our room and the first comment she made was how the energy in our room was so bright and uplifting. She said that she just came from the room down the hall where it was just the opposite, full of gloom. In this situation, it can be very easy to get lost in depression. I often found myself teetering on the edge of it. It made me think of that woman and her son and I wondered whether that was the room the chaplain was referring to. Truth be told, I never liked these visits from the chaplain. I associated her with some scary thoughts. I know she was there to provide support, but whenever she came, my thoughts went to some dark places that I never want to visit. I can't even bring myself to write it. In my mind, the chaplain is the last person you want to see at a hospital.

Being in that wing was very difficult and very surreal, but we did our best to make sure that Maddy never felt our worries, our sadness, or our fears. Trust me, we had plenty of them, but our priority was to make it as happy a place as we could for our son, despite the circumstances. Creating a cheerful environment was good for him and it was good for us. Sometime, maybe days later, I saw that woman I was talking about, the one with the teenage son, in the hallway. This time, there was something very different about her. I noticed and felt it right away. Her energy was different. Her face wasn't sunken with the sadness that I usually saw. This time, she looked happy. I saw HOPE. After several days of quietly passing each other in the hallway, our eyes met and we smiled at each other for the first time. No words, just a smile between two mothers that love their sons so very much. It was just a brief moment in time, but we made a connection. Later that day, I found out that her son was being released and that they were finally headed home. Home. I was so happy for her, for them. I may not know their story, but on that day, I knew that she had known happiness once again. It lightened my mood and made me eager for the day when we too would be headed home.

Chapter Sixteen

While we were at the hospital Maddy was placed on a heavy regimen of steroids as part of the Intensive Phase of his treatment. Some of the side effects of these steroids were extreme hunger, bloating in the face, and moodiness, all of which were expected to present itself fairly quickly. The funny thing was, several days went by and we hadn't noticed any of these side effects. Even the nurses were shocked and would ask me, "He's not hungry yet?" I mean of course he got hungry, but nothing out of the ordinary. Then, boom! After about a week and a half, the hunger came on like gangbusters. Maddox was ravenous all the time, at all hours of the day - and night! He ate tons of chicken tenders from the cafeteria, breakfast sausage from home, and cheese, lots and lots of cheese.

I have a very distinct memory of one night in particular. I was lying in bed next to him when sometime around two or three o'clock in the morning, Maddox starts yelling, "Cheese! Chicken!" He was very grumpy about it as the steroids can also cause irritability. Trust me, hunger and grouchiness are not a good combination, especially in the wee hours of the night. Well, we didn't have any chicken tenders, but we did have a whole pack of sliced cheese. Half asleep, I peeled myself out of bed, got the cheese from the fridge, and got back in bed with Maddy. I remember laying there in the dark, very groggy and tired, with Maddox next to me, his lips smacking and chomping slice after slice of cheese until the whole pack was gone. I must admit, despite my exhaustion, it was really quite amusing.

On another occasion, Maddox was really craving those breakfast sausage links. I usually made tons of them ahead of time at home to bring to the hospital, but we must have ran out, and the cafeteria did not have them as it was around dinner time. Well, Maddy was not pleased. He kept screaming for sausage. "Sausage! I want sausage!" I couldn't calm him down. I offered him all sorts of snacks and food, but all he wanted was sausage. I called home as I wasn't sure what else to do. So Cathie made what was probably two packages of breakfast sausage and walked it all the way to the hospital which by the way, was a little over a mile walk each way. When she got there with a container full of this precious meat, Maddox was satiated and I was so relieved! That kid ate sausage all night long.

On a different note, there was one afternoon that Maddox really wanted those chicken tenders from the cafeteria. I didn't want to leave him alone in the room to go and get them. It was around this time that Maddox's grandpa, Dave, arrived to support our family and to be with his wife. Cathie had come the day after Maddy was admitted to the hospital so it had been a while since Dave and Cathie had seen each other and I'm sure they were missing each other. Dave and Cathie were with Danika at the playground across the street from the hospital so Dave offered to get the chicken tenders from the cafeteria. Up until this point, Dave had not seen Maddy since Maddy was admitted into the hospital. When he came to the door holding a cup full of chicken tenders, Maddox was so excited to see him, and with a big smile said, "Hi Grandpa!" Dave saw his grandson for the very first time sitting there in his hospital tiger pajamas and quite suddenly, this very tall, stern, and imposing man, with tears in eyes, got very choked up. At 6'5, Dave can appear to be a very intimidating man. His voice broke and he looked down as he said, "Hi Maddy." It caught me off guard as I had never seen my father-in-law like this. He couldn't even bear to stay and quickly left after handing me the chicken. Thinking about it now, I guess I should have ran after to him to make sure that he was okay, but at the time, it just seemed like he didn't want me, or his grandson, or anyone for that matter, to see him like that. Witnessing Dave's reaction to Maddy being in the hospital made me very emotional as well. This was effecting all of us so very deeply. That was the only time I ever saw my father-in-law turn into a pile of mush. That was tough.

Chapter Seventeen

As the days at the hospital came and went, we did our best to make the time go by. Brad brought his laptop and was able to get some work done, I surfed the internet and even did some occasional online shopping, Maddy spent most of his days watching PBS Kids or *Blues Clues* on DVD, and Cathie brought Danika to the nearby playground and to the hospital to visit Maddy almost every day. The Child Life staff often came with games or toys for the kids.

When I look at some of the pictures we took at the hospital, it all seemed so ordinary, when in reality it was anything but. There is this one picture in particular of Brad and me that I look at with amazement. We are sitting together and I have this big smile on my face. So does Brad. The smiles didn't look forced or laced with sadness. It looked genuine and real. I honestly don't know how we got to the point where we could smile like that again. Yet, there it was. Somehow, we found a way to cope.

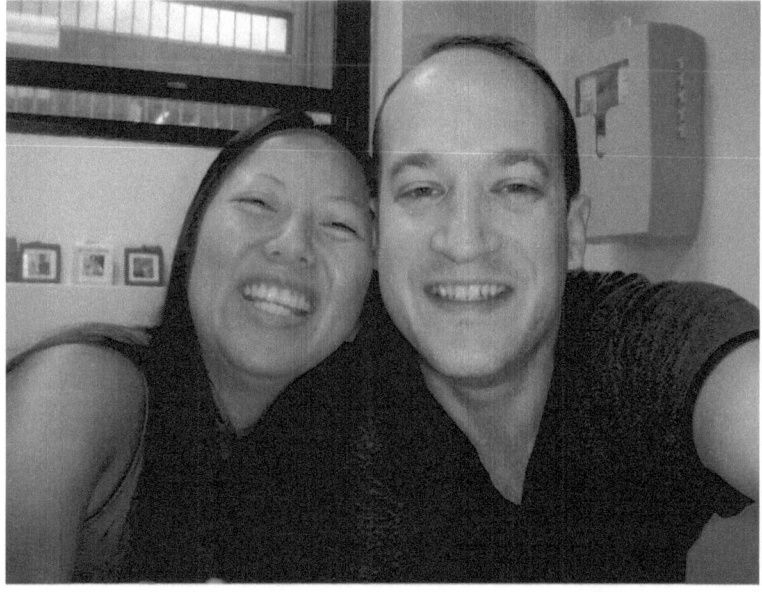

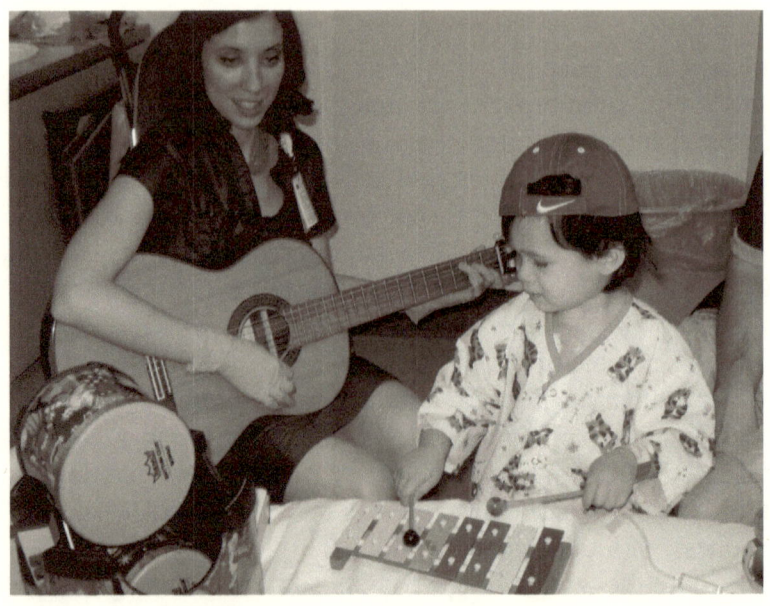

The wonderful Child Life program at Mount Sinai Hospital.

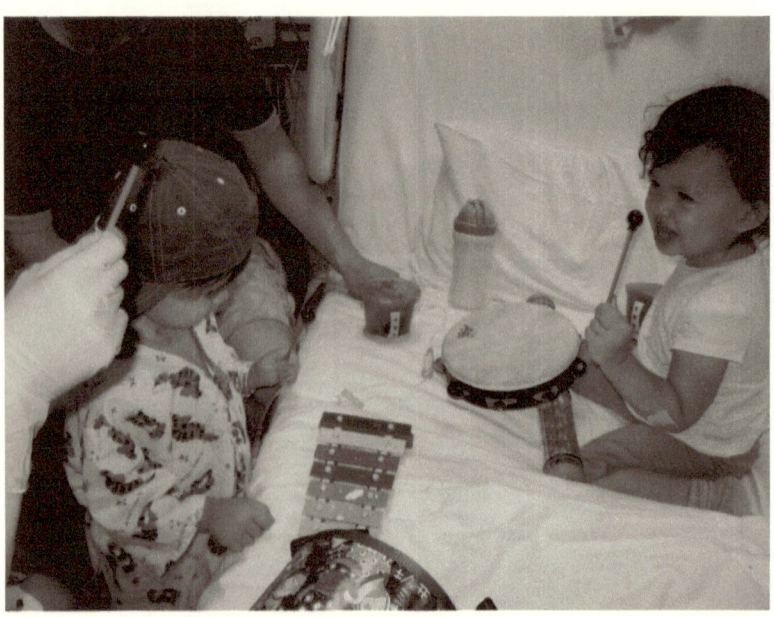

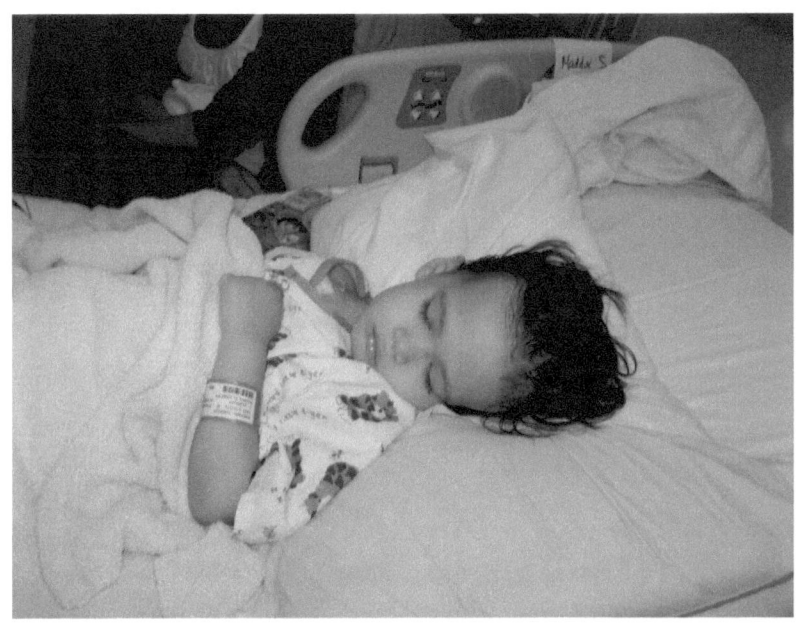

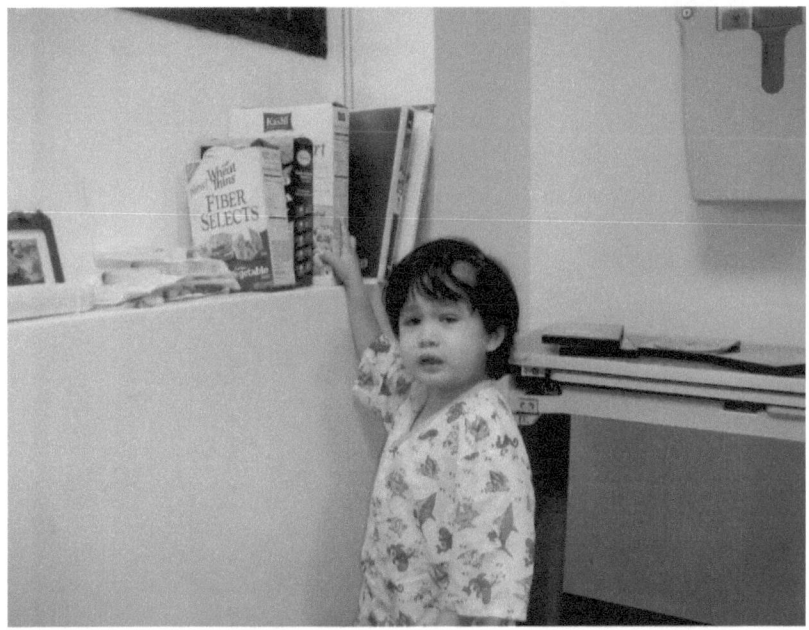

Maddox on steroids - literally.

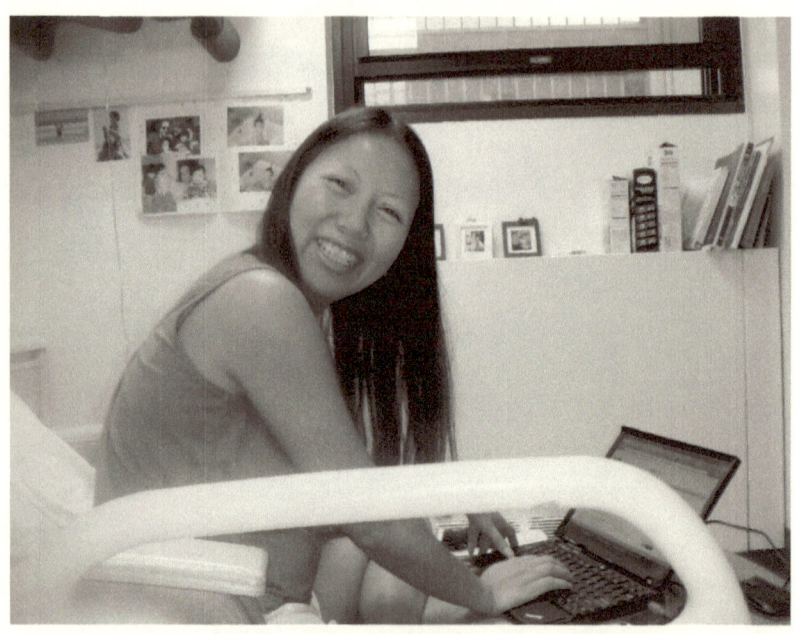

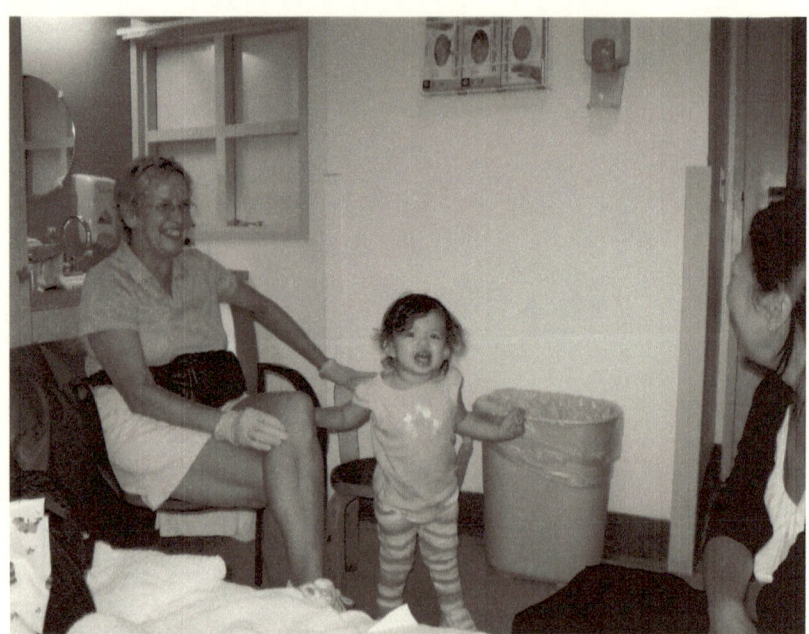

Grandma Cathie and Danika visit us at the hospital.

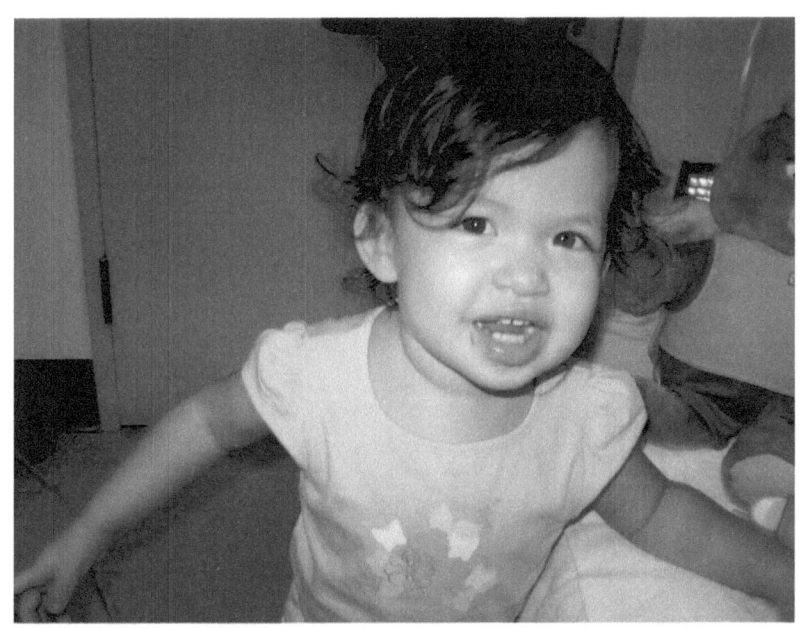

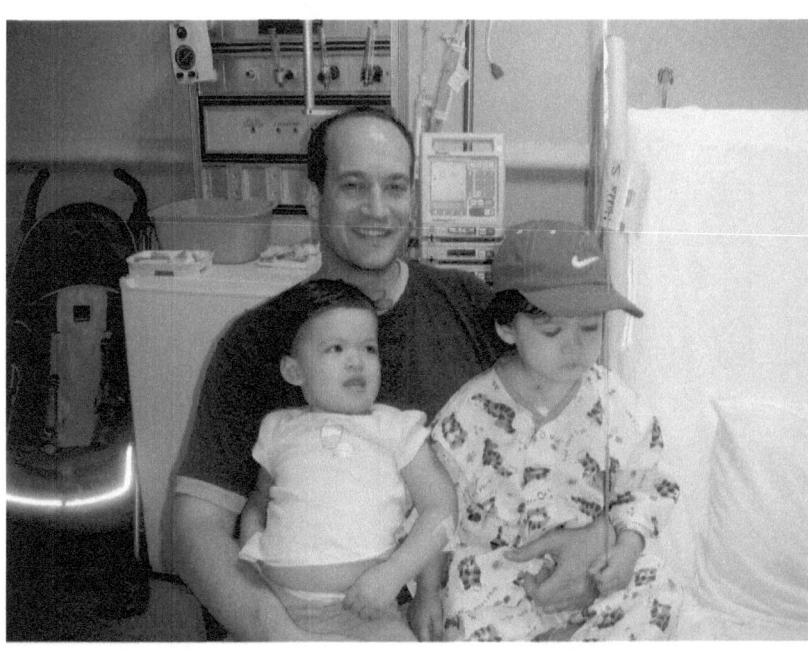

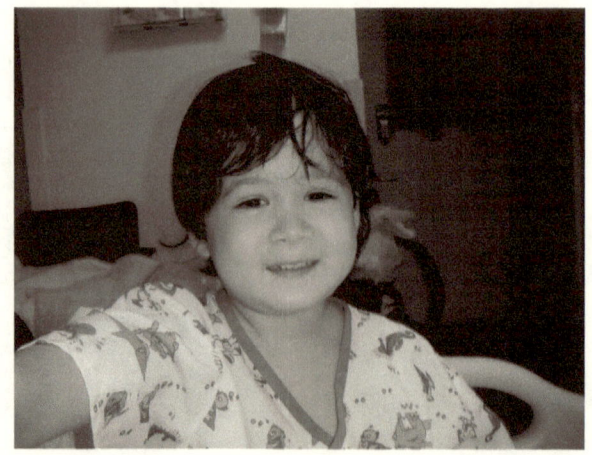

Our Brave Maddy.

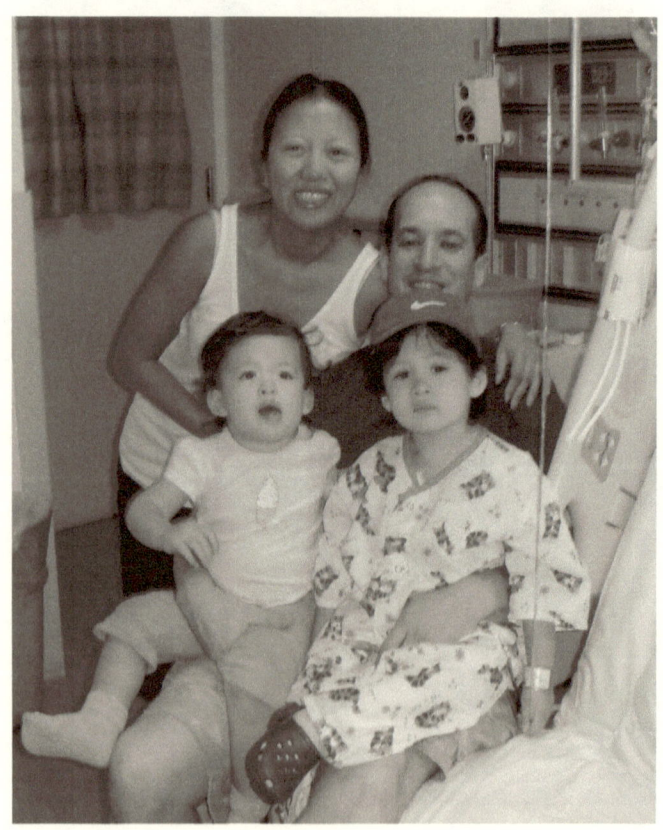

Chapter Eighteen

After a few weeks of treatment, Maddy was scheduled to take a test to make sure that the chemo was working. This was a very big deal. I remember the night I got the results. I was with Maddy at the hospital and Brad was home with Danika and his parents. The lights were dim in the room. Maddox was sleeping and I was lying on the pull-out chair bed just resting. All was quiet when I hear a light tap on the door as it is gently opened by Dr. Del Toro. I sit up with great anticipation. With the lights from the hallway shining into the room, I held my breath waiting as Dr. Del Toro says, "Mrs. Shepard, Maddox is in remission." In an instant, I felt myself collapse as all the built up tension was released from my body. I could breathe again. I exhaled out the biggest sigh of relief and began to cry - this time, tears of pure joy. I whispered, "Thank you, God." I sat there for a couple of minutes just taking in this good news, this GREAT, FANTASTIC news!

Maddox is in Remission!!!

I wanted some form of human contact to celebrate and mark this meaningful moment so I asked Dr. Del Toro if I could give him a hug, and before he could respond, I was up so fast and hugging him with all the thanks I had to give. After Dr. Del Toro left the room, I laid down next to Maddox and whispered softly in his ear, "You did it Maddy. You did it." With overwhelming gratitude in my heart, I just held him close to me, kissing him gently as he slept. My brave, brave little boy. I was so proud of him. After a short while, I called Brad at home and shared the good news with him. That was our first ray of light and we let it shine bright. We knew we still had a long road ahead of us, but now there was light to lead our way.

Chapter Nineteen

After weeks of intensive chemo treatment and isolation at the hospital, Maddy was discharged to continue his treatment at home, with clinic visits as scheduled. The day he was released, my favorite nurse, Raj went over all of the medicines and chemo with me, teaching me how to administer them. I had paid attention to the routine while we were at the hospital, but I was always the observer. It would now be my responsibility to care for my son at home.

On Maddox's discharge day, I watched Raj show me all the gear which included masks, gloves, and various size syringes depending on the dosage of each medication. The masks and gloves were for my protection as I was to be handling the chemo. She showed me all the pills and explained how to crush them and mix them with water or juice. Maddox was too young to take the pills as is and some were too large for him to swallow so it was necessary to have the pills crushed and mixed with a liquid. There were other medicines that would be given in liquid form and she showed me how to properly measure them. In addition to that, there were even more medicines that were to be given in conjunction with the chemo in order to protect Maddox from the possible side effects of some of the drugs. We would be given a monthly calendar called a roadmap which would guide us so that we knew what chemo or drug Maddy got on specific days. This calendar would also note the dates Maddox was scheduled for certain procedures, as well as the dates Maddy would be given chemo through an IV at the clinic.

I listened carefully to everything and as she continued on with the "lesson," I realized that this was now all on me. I didn't want to panic, but I was scared. What if I gave him the wrong dose? What if I messed up the days he gets certain drugs? What if I forget to give him his chemo? All of these concerns whirled in my head. As much as I was so thankful and happy to be leaving the hospital, I wasn't exactly thrilled at the thought that I was now in charge of my son's treatment at home. Was I prepared for this responsibility??? As it turns out, I was not. How could any mother possibly prepare themselves for giving chemo to their child? The answer is, you just can't. It was horrific that I had to. In the weeks ahead I would experience just how daunting and overwhelming this task would be. No one signs up for this, but I would do everything I could to rise up to the challenge. In a very short time, I had to learn to be a nurse. As a parent there is no training for that. I would have to learn on the job and that's exactly what I did.

Chapter Twenty

Once I completed my crash course with Raj, we were set to leave the hospital. We packed up everything that made that room our home for the past several weeks. We took all the pictures down, we gathered all the toys and stuffed animals, and we changed Maddy from his hospital pajamas to his own clothes. In spite of my apprehension about having to give Maddy his chemo, it felt so good to be going home. We said our goodbyes and thank you's to all the nurses and staff and then we were out the door. The kids were safe in their strollers and then there we were, our whole family, walking home in the bright sunshine. It was over a mile walk to our apartment, but we didn't mind. All we cared about was that we were all together. We still remember making the turn on our street, walking towards our building and hearing Maddox gleefully say, "almost home," his real home, our family home. It felt wonderful to walk into our apartment all together. We, along with his younger sister Danika, welcomed Maddox home just in time for his third birthday. This was the best gift we all could have gotten.

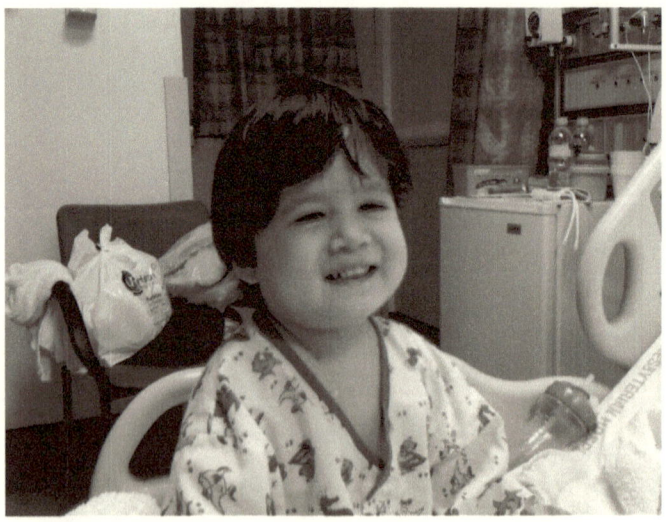

Maddy is discharged from the hospital!

I don't remember much more about that day except for this one moment. After getting settled back at home, I was sitting on the couch just watching Maddox. He was sitting on the floor and he was struggling to get himself up. It surprised me at first. Then it made me realize even more just how long we were at the hospital. I knew his leg muscles must have been weak from the lack of exercise. He had also gained some weight from the steroids. These steroids made him appear a bit bloated, especially in the cheeks. There he was, with his adorable baby face and chipmunk cheeks getting his bearings. My heart ached to look at him doing his best to get up - which he eventually did, but you could tell that it took some effort. At the hospital, Maddy spent most of his days just sitting or laying in bed. The room wasn't very big so he couldn't do much walking around in there. Since he was placed in isolation, he wasn't able to go to the playroom or even take a walk in the hallway. That hospital stay obviously took a toll on his body and he would now have to regain his strength. It made me even more thankful to finally be home where Maddy can run around and play and resume some sense of normalcy. Normalcy. That would be an interesting concept for us, especially after the past several weeks. We would soon have to redefine what that meant for our family. Later that day, Brad's work sent what must have been 20 - 30 celebratory balloons. The delight on Maddox and Danika's faces made that day even more special. We were finally home.

Several days later, we had a party to celebrate Maddox's Third Birthday. In the morning, right before the party, we all went for a walk in Central Park. One of the drugs Maddy had to take was Bactrim. He took this twice a day every Monday to Wednesday. One of the precautions while taking this drug was to avoid excessive sunlight. It was a gorgeous summer day in July so I remember we bought this huge sun shade canopy to put over Maddy's stroller to protect him from the sun. As careful as we could be, we set off for a leisurely stroll in the park. During the early part of his treatment, this was one of the few things we were able to do outside with Maddox. Going for strolls at Central Park became our connection to the outside world. Since his outside activities were limited, these casual walks became much welcome additions to our daily routine. Some days I would just park the double stroller next to a bench by the pond and the kids and I would look at the ducks or just watch those miniature remote control boats in the water. On the weekends, Brad and I would pack snacks for the kids and off we went to explore and discover parts of the park that we had never seen before. It was all we could really do so we took full advantage of it.

When Maddox was in the hospital, I would walk along Fifth Avenue, right next to Central Park on my way to and from the hospital, but never in these walks did I feel connected to the activities around me. On my walks to the hospital, all I wanted was to get there quickly to take care of my son. On my walks home, all I wanted was to get some rest and be there for my daughter. It was like I had tunnel vision oblivious of all the people, families, and children enjoying the park. I forced myself to ignore all of it because it was too painful to think about what we were missing. To be able to take these walks now was a beautiful thing. It felt good to be a part of it. It felt good to be a part of the world again.

There was one occasion, however, that I can recall when one of our walks in the park left me feeling disconnected once again. It was a beautiful sunny day and we must have already walked several miles when we came across a very festive scene. From a distance, it looked like some sort of carnival. The closer we got, the more I realized it was an amusement park. I later learned that it was a place called, Victorian Gardens, and up until that moment, I never even knew it existed. For a split second I thought, "How wonderful!" Then just as instantly, my heart sank and a sadness crept over me knowing that my kids couldn't be a part of it. From where I stood, I saw colorful rides and lots of children and their families smiling and having fun. Thinking back on that day, I have a distinct memory of facing the stroller away. I didn't want the kids to see it because I knew that we couldn't go. I hated the thought of having to disappoint them. They were already being deprived of so much of their childhood while Maddox was in treatment, I didn't want to add this to the list.

We probably should have turned away and kept on walking, but Brad and I stopped to watch. To me, it felt like we were outsiders looking in. It was right in front of us, within our reach, but our reality prevented us from just running in there. Thankfully, the kids were busy munching on their snacks unaware of it all. I looked longingly at this joyful place in front of me wishing that things were so very different, but they weren't. Maddy was still in the Isolation Phase and while he was cleared to go outside, exposing him to those crowds and the potential germs on the rides was just not an option.

It was so early on during his treatment that it was not easy to look beyond that point, but nevertheless, in the safest, deepest part of my being, I vowed that some day we too would get to enjoy that amusement park. It was this silent promise that allowed me to shake off the envy and the sadness and simply press onward. Instead of dwelling on what we couldn't do, I redirected my energy into appreciating that we were not in the hospital anymore. We were outside on a beautiful summer day. One small victory at a time. That's how we would get through this.

In the weeks ahead we must have covered every inch of Central Park. While we couldn't stop to have Maddox play on the grass or go on the swings, it was great to be out and about in nature and the open air.

Anyway, back to Maddy's birthday! On this special day, it was wonderful for all of us to get out of the house and enjoy the sights and sounds of the park. It may have come with some restrictions, but we were incredibly thankful for this freedom. After taking full advantage of the fresh summer air, we headed back home to get ready for Maddox's birthday celebration. Since Maddox was still supposed to be isolated from other children and visitors, it was a small party with just Brad, Danika, Grandma Cathie, and me as the guests. It was as happy a party as if there were 100 guests. Maddox got his first Thomas the Train set. This would be the first of many, many train sets. He would go on to collect and play with these trains for hours and hours. It was like Maddox's security blanket. Little did we know at the time that this toy would become

Maddox's main comfort on some pretty tough days. It gave our son joy during a difficult time, making it the best present ever. In a way I feel like this simple little tank engine took this journey with us. On this birthday, to watch the glee on Maddox's face as he said, "choo, choo," over and over again was priceless. For a brief moment, we forgot about the leukemia. In this moment, we simply enjoyed our little boy celebrating his birthday, being a regular kid, playing with a new toy. There were balloons, cake, presents, and a whole lot of love. We all had so much to be thankful for.

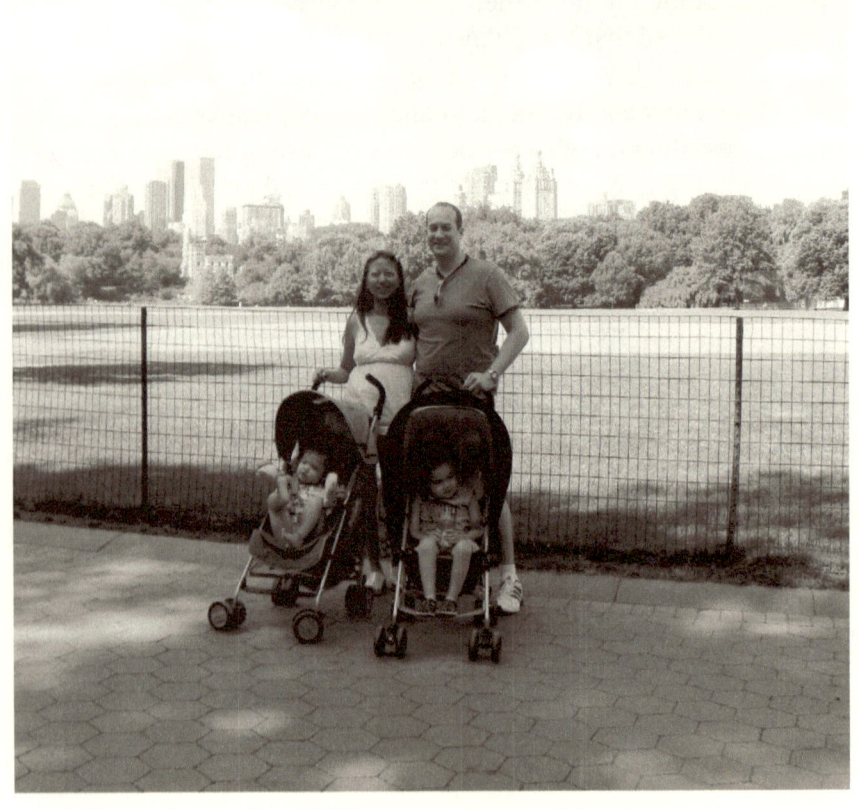

Beautiful Central Park.

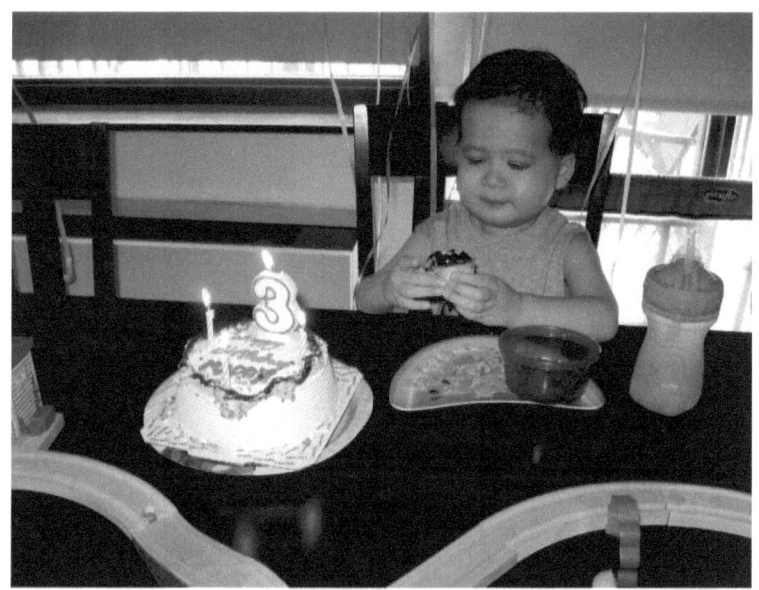

Happy Third Birthday, Maddox!

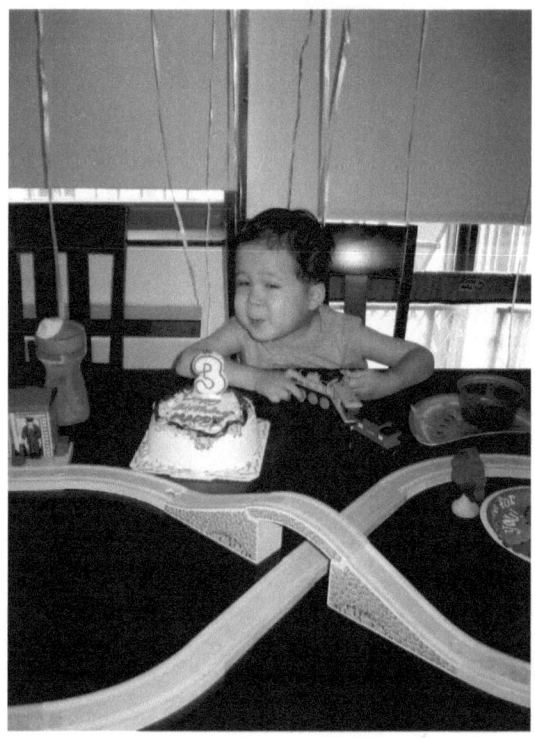

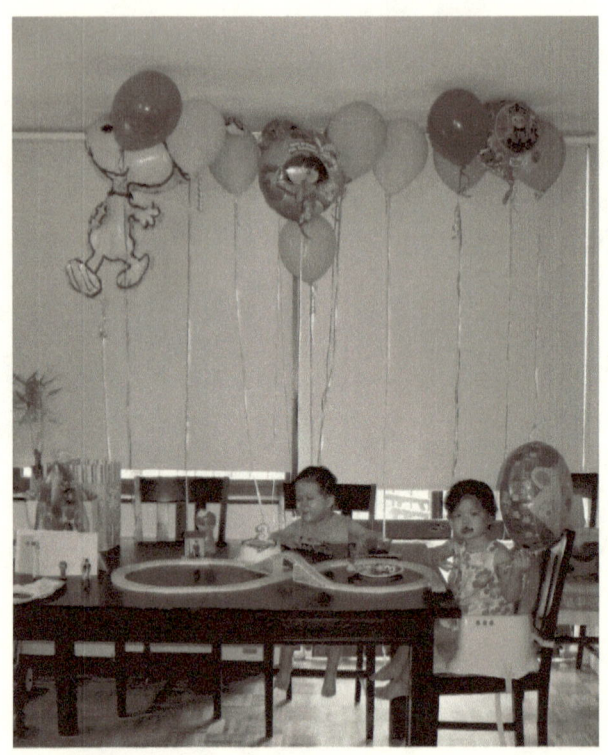

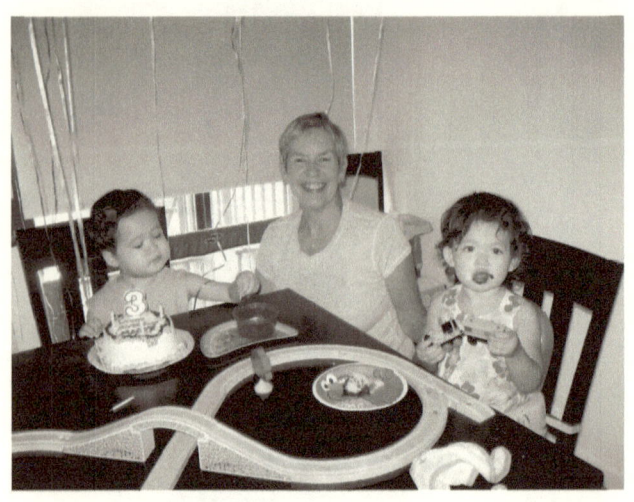

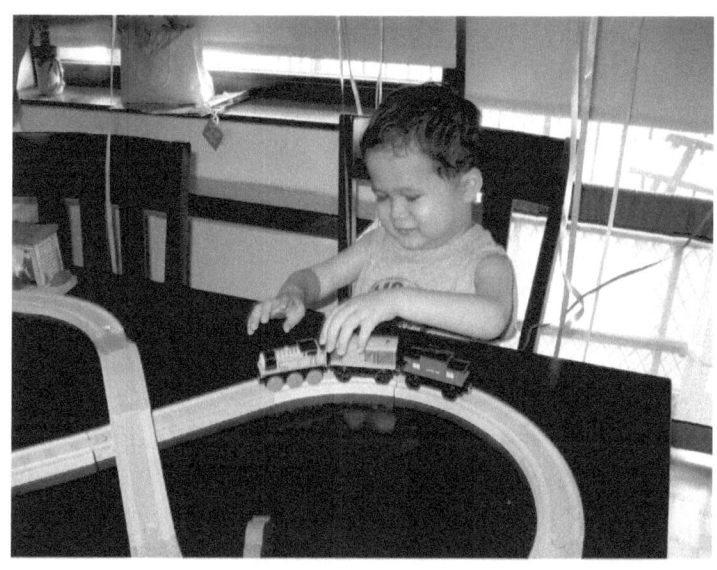

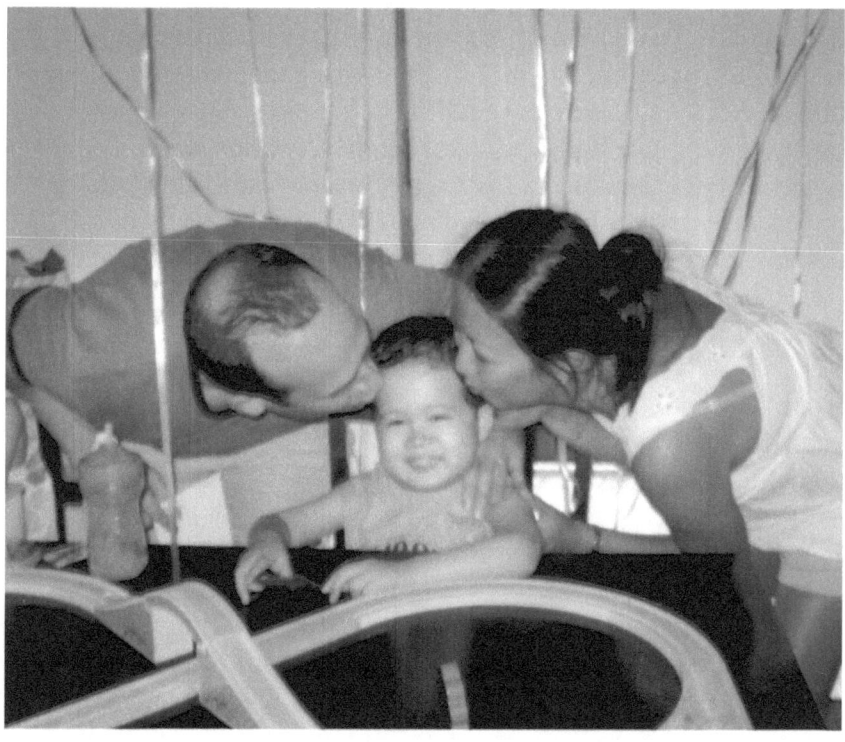

Chapter Twenty-One

One of the common side effects of chemo is hair loss. While we were at the hospital, we were told to prepare ourselves for when Maddox's hair started falling off. In fact, it was suggested that we get Maddox's head shaved in order to spare us the emotional trauma of watching our son's hair come out in clumps. Interestingly though, similar to the hunger with the steroids, Maddy did not experience this side effect right away. It should have started falling out while we were still at the hospital as that is when he began the Intense Phase of his treatment. I remember saying to myself that I would shave his head once I noticed his hair falling out. I just couldn't bring myself to shave it until then. Well days passed and nothing. I must say that it baffled many of the hospital staff. For me, it was a very welcome surprise because I knew that watching my son's hair fall out would devastate me. His bald head would be a constant, visible reminder of the cancer he was fighting. With hair, Maddy looked like any other "normal" kid. Once his hair fell off, there would be physical proof that my son was far from normal. Once the hair was gone, there for all the world to see, would be my sweet little boy undergoing chemo. That being said, it was kind of amazing that Maddox was discharged from the hospital with a full head of hair. He was at home, weeks into the heaviest chemo phase, and his hair was holding strong. It was really quite remarkable. It seems strange to say this, but I felt a sort of pride at this feat, that somehow, my son's body was stronger than the chemo.

On one of Maddy's clinic appointments, I remember one of the pediatric oncologists walking down the hallway looking at Maddox incredulously as she said, "I can't believe it. I don't think his hair is going to fall off." All I could do was be amused at her astonishment. A part of me was foolish enough to think that maybe, just maybe, it wouldn't fall off. Well, it wasn't long after that appointment that the inevitable happened. One morning, as I went to pick Maddox up from his crib, there on his pillow were clumps of hair. I gasped and thought, "Oh, no." I allowed myself a moment of shock as tears began to form in my eyes. I quickly shook it off. I could not, would not, let myself get lost in this moment, so I forced myself to bottle up my emotions before I let any tears fall. I quickly cleaned up the hair. I didn't want Maddox to see it even though at his young age he probably wouldn't have even understood, much less cared. I know I promised myself that I would shave his head at the first sign of his hair falling out, but I just couldn't do it. Each day after that, there would be more hair on his pillow. When I brushed his hair, strands and strands would just slide right off, and with every brush, I would suppress the sadness I felt. I know it seemed like I was torturing myself when I should have just shaved it, but I guess in a way, my refusal to shave it was really me desperately hanging on to this bit of "normal."

While I didn't shave it, I did cut - what was left of his hair - shorter. That I could do. Eventually though when you looked at Maddy's hair, all you could see were small sections or wisps just barely covering his scalp, until one day there was no hair left. I thought about what people would think when they saw my son. I hated that they would look at us and feel sorry for us. Then I thought, "To hell with that!" My son's bald head would be a badge of his COURAGE! As emotional as it was to make peace with it, I knew it was part of our journey. He may have been bald, but he was also very beautiful and very, very brave.

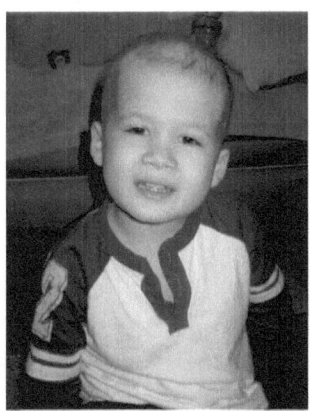

Chapter Twenty-Two

Once we were settled at home, there were various precautions we had to take. Because of the chemo, Maddox's immune system was heavily suppressed so he had no way to fight off any illnesses. He was still in the Intense Phase of his treatment so while he was home, we had to continue to isolate him. We had to be careful not expose him to outside elements and other children. This meant he couldn't go to school, or the playground, or even have play dates. He couldn't swim in the ocean or a public pool. We were told to avoid any enclosed public places where there would be large crowds. Consequently, we were strongly advised not to go to restaurants, take the train or bus, or travel on a plane. To keep our home as sterile as possible, we took our shoes off at the door and instructed any visitors to do the same. We even installed a Purell dispenser by the door to make sure everyone's hands were clean when entering the apartment. My God, when I look back on it now, I honestly don't know how we did it. We had to adjust to a whole new way of living. Of course we followed all of these necessary precautions to protect our son, but at the same time, it broke our hearts. Maddox was only three years old and Danika was only one and a half years old. This was a time when they should have enjoyed being toddlers, going to the playground, making new friends, and having play dates, but they couldn't. Instead, they were forced to amuse themselves in what was at the time, our very small Manhattan apartment. Because Maddox couldn't go out, in order to keep him safe, we also kept Danika home. As a result, Maddox and Danika were each other's only friends.

Our daughter was so young when all this happened to her big brother. I hate that I have very little memories of playing with Danika at that age. I just hate it. The truth is, because of our unimaginable circumstances, Brad and I know we neglected our beautiful daughter. As unintentional as it was, it was not fair to her. Nothing about this was fair. It tears me up inside to think about it. While Maddox was at the hospital, Danika spent a lot of time with her grandma. She watched her mommy and daddy in and out of the apartment not understanding why. When we finally brought Maddy home, I'm sure most of our attention went to him and his care. Of course Brad and I did our best to show both of our children that we loved them very much, but during that time, I know that we focused more on Maddox. We had to. Danika has always been a very observant child so I know this must have impacted her. Even writing about this now all I want to do is hold her close and show her how very much I love her. Oh how I desperately, achingly, long for those days of playing with my sweet one year old girl before the cloud of cancer turned all of our lives upside down. I know every age is special when it comes to our children, but anyone who is a parent would agree when I say that there is just something so magical about your child when they are just one and two years old. At that age, they are so pure and innocent, and may even still have that delicious baby smell. Their giggles melt your heart. They are making discoveries every day and the wonder in their eyes is simply glorious. It breaks me a million times over to know that so many of those special Mommy moments were stolen from me, from all of us.

I know Danika sensed how much more attention was given to her brother. When I would leave her with Brad or a babysitter to take Maddox to the clinic, Danika always got very upset. She would cry and cry wanting to come with us. In her mind, the clinic was a place where children got to play with toys. How could we explain to her that we were there because her older brother was fighting a very serious illness. Danika thought we were taking Maddox to some place fun, as if we were depriving her of something enjoyable. Little did she realize that the clinic was the very last place any of us wanted to be.

On some level, even at such a young age, Danika knew that something was different, that something just wasn't right. Her awareness became obvious to me on one particular occasion. It happened one day during those early weeks when we as a family were still trying to cope with Maddy's diagnosis. While Brad was with Maddy at the hospital, I took Danika to music class. Prior to that, we had Cathie taking her so that both Brad and I could be at the hospital with our son. I knew it was important for me to spend time with my daughter, so that morning, Danika got some time with her mommy, something that was becoming a rarity. The class was called the Music Room and Maddox and Danika loved singing and dancing to Teacher Paul's music. A week earlier, it was Cathie that told Teacher Paul why Maddox wasn't in class, so when he saw me that day for the first time since hearing of Maddox's diagnosis, he gave me a look of compassion and understanding. He came up to me and said that he would love to go to the hospital to play his guitar and sing for Maddox. Incredibly touched by his kind offer and words of support, I began to tear up. Struggling to keep my composure, I thanked him and explained that we were under strict orders to limit visitors while Maddox was in isolation. He replied that he would be happy to come anytime. It was such a thoughtful gesture and made me realize even more how many people cared about our son.

During the class, I did my best to be completely there with my daughter, but a part of me was at the hospital thinking about Maddox. This was so not fair to Danika, but despite my best efforts to be truly present for her, I found my attention split in two different places.

At the end of the class, some of the kids liked to give Teacher Paul a quick hug before leaving. On this day, for Danika, it was anything but quick. I watched her tentatively walk up to him and quietly wait until it was her turn. With Teacher Paul kneeling down to reach her level, Danika put her head on his shoulders and placed her arms around him and just stayed there - for a really long time. She literally clung on to him for a good three to four minutes. Being the kind man that he was, he never once tried to break free. He knew that my little girl needed some comfort. I watched this display of affection willing the tears not to fall. My heart was breaking. It was as if Danika was clinging on to him in an effort to cling on to better days when she and her brother were there together. It seemed like she was desperate to hang on to something, *anything* that was "normal" and familiar. She was just a baby, barely able to express herself, but in that simple moment, her actions spoke volumes. It became very clear to me, that like the rest of us, Danika was hurting too. It tortures me to think about how much both my son and daughter sacrificed of their childhoods.

While this story centers around Maddy, it is important to acknowledge what my beautiful daughter, Danika, gave up to help take care of her big brother. For many weeks, we didn't take her to the playground for fear that she may catch something and then expose Maddox to it. For the same reasons, we didn't let her go on any play dates either. We were cautious about everything because we were so scared of Maddy getting sick. Even a common cold was his enemy. In our efforts to protect him, we deprived Danika of so many fun activities that every child should enjoy. We stopped going to the Music Room with Teacher Paul. I stopped taking Danika to those "Mommy and Me" classes, and we didn't even allow her to go to any of those play gyms afraid of what germs she many bring into the apartment. Danika lost so much of that wonderful time and she didn't even know it. Children adapt so quickly that gradually, staying at home with Maddy, just became what was normal to her.

We later discovered that this "seclusion" would have a huge effect on Danika socially. She became very shy and anxious whenever there were new people around. I know this is not unusual for most kids, but what made Danika's behavior a concern was that she not only became shy, she also became somewhat fearful, even around family. I remember one day when her Uncle Todd and Uncle Said came to visit, Danika spent the whole time hiding under the dining room table. We literally could not get her to come out. This was not the playful and outgoing Danika we knew. She had changed. Her behavior became the product of our incredible circumstances.

I have a vivid memory of a day when we were at the playground. This was after Maddy was done with isolation and it was okay for us to go to the playground again. I remember that Danika sat herself next to three girls who were playing together. I noticed Danika just watching them. She didn't try to join them in their play or even talk to them, and the girls were too involved in each other to notice Danika sitting right beside them. Danika just sat quietly next to them until the three girls got up and ran to another activity. She did not follow them, but instead ran up to me excitedly and said, "Mommy, I made new friends!" It was such a bittersweet moment for me. It was wonderful to see my daughter so happy, but at the same time, my heart sank when I realized that that is what Danika thought it meant to make new friends. In her mind, just being in their presence made them all friends. She was so proud of herself. I didn't want to take that joy away from her, so with the same excitement I said, "That's great, Dan!" I wanted her to feel good about herself. I may have at some point encouraged her to go after those girls and play with them, but for Danika, just having sat beside them was enough for her and so in that moment, it was enough for me.

Brad and I truly believe that not having those play dates and not going to those toddler classes really effected Danika's ability to socialize. Basically, Maddox was Danika's one and only play date for those months that Maddy was in isolation. She didn't have the opportunity to learn how to make friends, or be part of activities with other toddlers, or just in general be exposed to other people and children. Because of that, she really didn't get a chance to develop any social skills. For a very long time, all she knew was us. Her comfort was just us - her mommy, her daddy, and Maddy.

There was another significant factor that came into play as well. I strongly believe it is the root of a lot of Danika's fears. I'm no psychologist, but I think it also has to do with the fact that out of no where, all of a sudden, it was her grandma taking care of her. This was during those early weeks when Maddox was in the hospital. As a little baby, it must have been so confusing for her that one minute we, her parents, were there with her all the time, and then the next moment, we were in and out of our apartment, barely there, with grandma being her only constant. She must have wondered why her brother wasn't home playing with her and why her mommy and daddy looked so sad and worried. Her family was being torn apart.

Of course Brad and I did our best to protect and shield Danika from what was going on, but the pain was too raw. As much as we tried to "fake it until we make it" for the sake of our daughter, I am sure the reality of our situation was written all over our faces. During those early weeks, the mood in our apartment was heavy. She knew something was terribly wrong, but how could such a little child possibly process all of that. Gradually, Danika began to withdraw. I guess by sheltering herself from others, Danika found a way to cope, and perhaps escape. Whenever there was someone at the door, Danika would immediately run to her room, or if we made her stay, Danika would fiercely cling on to me or Brad. I think she associates any visitors with what happened with her grandma. Cathie came to our home and was basically the one who took care of her while Brad and I spent most of our time at the hospital. It must have seemed like we just abandoned her. This fear of abandonment is probably what caused Danika to retreat whenever we had any company. It is my belief that whenever anyone came to our house, Danika became terrified that Mommy and Daddy would leave her again to be taken care of by someone else.

It devastates me to think that my daughter had to handle these fears at such a delicate age. I have this video that I took of Maddox and Danika when it just their grandma and grandpa visiting us. Everyone was in the living room while Danika was in her and Maddy's bedroom, holding on tightly to the side of her crib. Her hair still had those cute baby curls that I love. I can hear myself in the video saying, "C'mon out Danika, it's okay." Then Maddox, in his sweet baby voice, would repeat what I said, trying to get his baby sister to come out, "Is okay, is okay, c'mon out Nika." Danika would look down and just shake her head no. Maddy would reach for her hand to try to get her to follow him, but she wouldn't budge, too scared to come out. I recently watched this video that was taken years ago and the heartache is no less. I'm overwhelmed with sadness whenever I think about this and what the events of those days did to our sweet baby girl.

I'm thankful to say that eventually, and with some time, Danika found her way back to being the playful, goofy, animated, and social daughter we know and love. While Maddox was in treatment, we all had to learn to adapt and adjust to a new way of living. Taking it one day at a time, slowly, slowly, we made our way out of the darkness and into the light, determined as a family to survive it all. Gradually, some "normalcy" came back in our lives, and with that, Danika found comfort and security in our home and our family once again. The most important thing to know is that Danika gained her confidence back and that made all the difference in the world - to all of us.

Chapter Twenty-Three

During those first difficult weeks following Maddox's diagnosis, Brad and I felt an overwhelming sense of helplessness. We were emotionally broken. I blamed myself for not being more proactive all those times we took Maddy to the pediatrician with fevers and various odd symptoms. I should have demanded answers and insisted that they take a closer look. I also blame the pediatrician's office for seriously dropping the ball. We were there enough times to warrant a more extensive examination of my son's condition. It should not be surprising that we later switched to another pediatrician. There were so many thoughts that went through our heads. Brad and I questioned and agonized over and over again whether there was something we did that caused this, or whether there was something we didn't do that could have prevented this from happening, when the truth of the matter is - there is no known definitive cause. In order to move on and move forward we would just have to accept that, and eventually, we did. To get through this, we knew that we had to put away all the blame and all the guilt. Once we recovered from the shock if it all, we did our best not to think about what we couldn't change, but instead focused our energy on all the things we could do to get our son well.

The outpouring of love and support for our family was truly moving. Meals showed up at our door regularly, toys were constantly arriving, months worth of complimentary maid service was given to keep our home clean, and a couple of friends even fasted for a week as part of their prayers - so amazing. We were told many times to "stay strong." This would have been almost impossible had it not been for the strength and courage of our son and the love of our family and friends.

Every once in a while, out of nowhere, while simply walking down the block or just watching some random TV program, the reality of our situation would hit me and I would find myself struggling to fight off all the emotions. I didn't like being in that place so each day I did my best to focus on the good. Despite everything he has endured, Maddy continued to be a happy, sweet, and loving child.

Maddox absolutely loved playing with Thomas the Train and is quite a musical child who loves to sing, dance, and play instruments. During the early months of his treatment, Maddy enjoyed his favorite shows, *Blues Clues, Super Why,* and *Sesame Street,* just to name a few. Watching Maddox perform the theme song to *Blues Clues* brought smiles to our faces every time. In fact, we have a great video of Maddy mimicking the host, singing the theme song to the show, to a tee. To look at him you'd never know the hell he's been through. It's Maddy's laughter that magically made it all better and it is his joy that gave us courage. We knew that we had quite a road ahead of us, but with the support of our family and friends, we took it one day at a time, drawing strength from all the love that surrounded our family. That is what would get us through the next three and a half years. We were counting on it.

Chapter Twenty-Four

The Routine

Getting settled at home with a whole new routine absolutely had its challenges.

The Medicine

As part of his treatment, Maddy would get chemo and other supportive drugs at home, by mouth through a syringe. The chemo was a pill called mercaptopurine or 6MP. I would crush this pill and mix it with juice because it was too big for Maddy to swallow. Once the pill was mixed, I would draw it into a syringe and squeeze it into Maddox's mouth. This juice mixture is what I would do for all the drugs that came in pill form. Every four weeks, Maddox was put on steroids called Decadron. He would take these steroids everyday, twice a day, for 5 days after he got IV chemo, called vincristine at the hospital. To prevent any stomach irritation that the Decadron may cause, it was given with Zantac which came in liquid form. Maddox was also on Bactrim, another liquid medicine, every Monday to Wednesday and later, it became every Monday to Thursday. He took this twice a day, once in the morning and again after dinner. On Thursdays, he took a drug called methotrexate. These pills were tiny and Maddy had to take 6 or 7 them to get the instructed dosage. I remember often checking myself, and meticulously counting these little pills over and over again to make sure that I got the right amount before I crushed them. I was so scared that I'd give him too many or not enough. The dosages sometimes changed with the 6MP and methotrexate. Whenever that happened, I had to be careful to cut some of the pills in half so that I administered the correct dose.

On some occasions, when Maddox's counts dipped below a certain level, usually due to a fever or some infection he caught, we had to stop the chemo all together. This would allow Maddy's body a chance to recover. On the one hand, it was a nice break not to have to prepare the chemo for several days, but on the other hand, I was so afraid of what would happen if we kept him off the chemo for too long. After all, it is the chemo that kills the cancer. As much as I hated giving it to him, I knew it was our best weapon against this horrible disease. There was so much detail involved with understanding and administering these pills and in the beginning, I was completely overwhelmed, terrified that I would screw it up. I was responsible for giving chemo to my son. My God, how could any parent ever wrap their head around that. It would prove to be a very daunting and extremely emotional task.

The Steroids

As part of his treatment, Maddox was put on a regimen of steroids called Decadron every four weeks. As I said, he would take it twice a day, once in the morning and then generally after dinner, for five days. The side effects of these steroids were truly a bitch, not just on Maddy, but on all of us. After a couple of days on it, Maddox's demeanor and disposition would range from fatigue and extreme hunger, to down right crankiness, bordering on mean. Through no fault of his own, Maddy would go through these extreme mood swings. One moment he'd be sad and mopey, and the next moment, he would be in a fit of anger over the littlest thing. How awful it must have been for him to be in such a state of emotional discomfort and not know why. I hated watching him go through these cycles. It was bad when he was cranky, but the toughest moments for me were when Maddox had no energy at all. Maddy would just simply lay down on the couch for hours. It was those moments that I'd be hit with such sadness. No parent wants to see their child in such a condition. In choosing the lesser of two evils, in some ways I preferred it when Maddy was cranky. At least then, there'd be some fire in him.

Maddox became a totally different person when he was on these drugs. It was already a challenge giving Maddox his chemo, but when he was on steroids, it took it to a whole other level. He not only resisted getting the medicine, but often went into a rage beyond the normal yelling and screaming that accompanied giving him his chemo. Those were some of the toughest days to give Maddox his medicine. It was not always easy, but during these Decadron cycles, we all did our best to make him as comfortable and as calm as we could. Only other parents who went through this would understand the toll it takes on the whole family and how steroids can transform a perfectly good natured child into a bit of a monster. It generally took about a week for the side effects of the steroids to wear off. Once it did, I got my sweet boy back.

Chapter Twenty-Five

I have so many painful memories of giving Maddox his chemo. To think about it now, all I want to do is make those memories go away. Every time he saw me with those syringes, he would run and cry. I couldn't blame him. Even mixed with juice, I know these pills must have tasted awful to him. During those first few months, it seemed like every day was an epic battle, especially when he was on those nasty steroids. Some days I literally had to hold him down on the couch to prevent him from hitting or kicking me so that I could get the syringe into his mouth. I would be crying, willing him to cooperate, and absolutely hating every moment that I had to restrain my own child. I couldn't believe that this was my reality. In between tears and utter helplessness, I would just beg for him to take his medicine saying, "Please Maddy, please, please."

I remember one time, in my desperation to give Maddy his chemo, while holding him down, with his arms and legs flailing about, I quickly squirted the syringe straight into his mouth, directly at his throat. To my horror, he immediately gagged it all out. He was yelling and crying the whole time. I was beside myself freaking out because one, he basically threw it all up and second, there was now chemo mixed with vomit all over Maddy and the floor. I didn't know whether it posed any danger for skin to come in contact with the chemo so I frantically cleaned Maddox and the floor up as quickly as I could, trying desperately to hold on to my sanity. There I was, sobbing, on my hands and knees, in the middle of this mess. Was this really my life? With Maddy crying in the background, I yelled at Danika, who was standing there watching me with a look of utter confusion, and screamed at her, "Stay back! Stay back!" I had to protect her. I didn't want her anywhere near this. Oh man, I was losing it. Danika must have wondered what the heck her mommy was doing to her big brother. What a scene that must have been for her. In a frenzy, after I completely sanitized the area, I called the clinic. I must have sounded like a crazy person telling the nurse what had happened. She calmly said that it was fine and then she told me that I had to give it to him again. Wait, what?!!! No effin' way!!! She explained that because he spit it out so quickly, none of it went into his system. No! No! No! Both my son and I were already traumatized and exhausted from these events. How in the world was I possibly going to do that again??? I must have blocked the memory out because I honestly can't remember how I did it. Somehow, some way, that boy got his chemo that day.

That would not be the only time Maddy would gag his chemo or medicine out. Each time it would leave me physically and emotionally drained. Having to restrain my son so that I can force him to take this poison took a huge toll on me. Some days I had to physically get on top of him to keep his arms and legs from hitting me. The strength and effort it took to hold him down and keep him steady, while at the same time making sure that I didn't hurt him, was more than I could bear. I remember far too many days when I would go to my room after giving Maddy his chemo and surrender to the loneliness I felt. In the privacy of my bedroom, I would just cry and cry and cry, praying, begging, for strength. Brad never knew the countless afternoons I wept in our bedroom after a physical, emotional, and mental battle with our son to make sure he got his chemo.

On one occasion, I asked Brad to give Maddy his medicine. I laid all the pills out, with the syringes and the pill crusher, and any other gear, along with instructions on the dosages. Shortly after Brad gave Maddy his chemo, I was putting all the bottles and gear away when I noticed that the number of pills left in one of the bottles did not make sense. To my horror, I realized that Brad must have combined two different pills together! Our son just ingested these pills! I feared that we gave him some dangerous concoction, that combining those two pills would somehow harm our son. In an instant, I went from zero to sixty. I was furious with Brad for making such a gross error. I was furious with myself that maybe my instructions were not clear enough. Brad was at the computer when I rushed into the room and told him what happened. I wanted to lash out at him, to accuse him, but something stopped me. Somehow I had the sense to know that if I had said all the things that I wanted to say, it would have taken us to a place where our relationship may not have been able to recover. Whatever instinct it was that stopped me, it probably saved our marriage. While I struggled to keep those urges under control, the rest of me lost it. I couldn't take it out on him, but boy I sure took it out on me. I started to unravel and with both of my hands curled into fists, I started hitting and literally punching my cheeks and forehead really hard, saying, "Oh my God! Oh my God!" It was as if I wanted to hurt or punish myself. I was hysterical. I had no idea how those two drugs would interact when mixed together. I was terrified of what it might do to our son. When Brad saw me hitting myself, I could tell by the look on his face that he knew I was over the edge and he looked scared. He grabbed my hands away from me to stop me from hurting myself as he tried to calm me down. We called the clinic together. The person who answered the phone must have heard the extreme panic in my voice because she put me straight through to the doctor on duty. I was crying uncontrollably at this point telling the doctor what had happened. She was quick to try to settle me down and reassured me that it was all okay. She said that the pills were all going into Maddox's system anyway so mixing the two different pills would not cause any harm. She went on to say that they would not give parents this responsibility if there were any serious safety concerns. While it all turned out okay, Brad and I realized that it was me that was *so* not okay. I had come undone. My reaction to hit myself scared both of us. It was very obvious that the stress of managing my son's chemo was getting to me. In my mind, if Brad helped more with giving Maddy his medicine, he would have known that those two pills look very different, and he would have known, *should* have known that they do not get mixed together. I strongly believed that it was his responsibility too to know what medicines Maddy took, but instead Brad relied on me to know everything. That was an enormous responsibility. It felt like I had the weight of the world on my shoulders. Whenever we were asked to provide Maddy's medical information, it was me that could recite the list of chemo and drugs without even thinking about it. I felt that my husband should be able to do the same. I was consumed with these thoughts, but I kept it all inside. Perhaps I should have confronted Brad about all of these feelings that day, but I guess I was afraid of where it would lead and I just did not have the energy to argue. I was already spent, too exhausted to feel anything except relief that Maddy was okay.

This is when I started to have some resentment towards Brad for not sharing the responsibility of giving Maddox his chemo. He became well aware of this resentment soon enough. We must have been arguing over something to do with Maddy's medicine when I finally told him how I felt. This topic often found it's way into several of our "talks." Sometimes we discussed it calmly, but most of the time, the issue was a hot button for both of us. I understood that he couldn't do it during the week because of work. Of course I know that is very important. Brad works very hard. He takes care of our family and I love him for that. I know he thinks that I don't have a true appreciation for how hard he works, but I really do. It's just that I needed some help. One day, I remember asking Brad if he could at least do Maddy's chemo on the weekends so that I could get a little break from it. His answer was simply that he preferred that I did it. Well that was that. I don't think he was being insensitive on purpose. I just think he felt more comfortable with me doing because I was already doing it. To be fair, Brad did step up many times when I occasionally asked him to do it, but for the most part, it was my "job." Whenever Brad did do it, I was usually there to help him hold Maddy when Maddy resisted taking the medicine. I was there to distract Maddy or calm him down. All the other times, except for perhaps the weekends, I was flying solo. If Maddy fought me, I had no one there to help me settle him down. When Maddy screamed and cried, I was the one that soothed him. I was the one who had to watch my son go through this torture every day. I envied Brad being at his job not having to suffer watching his son be subjected to this every day. Brad could get lost in his work, he could socialize with his coworkers, and maybe, just maybe, even for a brief second, he could be distracted enough to forget about what was happening in our lives. I did not have this luxury. Every time I put on those gloves and those masks, every time I laid out all the pills and the gear, and every single time that I braced myself to give my son chemo, I was reminded that my little boy was battling cancer. Having that responsibility every day never let me forget it.

Chapter Twenty-Six

The Fevers

Those were rough. Because of chemo, Maddox was more susceptible to germs and viruses. Whenever Maddox got a fever, it, more times than not, booked us a stay at the hospital. A big reason for this was to make sure that there was no infection from his port. Whatever the case may be, whether it was a virus or an infection, Maddox usually had to get antibiotics to protect him from whatever it was that was causing the fever. Should Maddox develop a fever before 5PM, we could take him directly to the clinic. After 5PM, we would have to take Maddox to the ER. The thing with the Pediatric ER for Mount Sinai was that it handled cases all across the board. It was not devoted to just children in treatment like the clinic. Because of that, it was always best to avoid the ER and go to the clinic. However, it just so happened that whenever Maddox developed a fever, it was almost always after 5PM. Go figure, huh. Brad and I were always like, "Aw c'mon!"

It was a rare occasion when Maddy got a fever during the day. On those rare days, here is generally how the day would play out. Maddy would wake up and just be out of sorts. He would either be really tired or he would have no appetite. I could always tell when he wasn't himself. The kids were usually always up early. I remember in the mornings, lying in bed, I would always be relieved to hear the sounds of activity and play from the kids. Whenever it was too quiet, I would know that something was probably up. Maddox is such a morning person so if he was still in bed, I knew something must be brewing. In some ways, these days were tougher to deal with compared to the days when he just straight up got a fever. One of the hardest things for me was the constant vigilance, waiting to find out whether Maddy would develop a fever. On these days, Brad usually got two phone calls at work. I would make the first call to him in the morning giving him the heads up that Maddox was not feeling well. This would give him a chance to coordinate things at work in case he had to abruptly head home. Then, I would make the second call, hours later, either telling him that all was well or telling him to come home so that one of us could take Maddox to the clinic. Brad never really knew what went on during the time he got the first call, to the time he got the second call.

Those hours waiting to find out whether Maddy would need to go to the clinic were not easy. For hours I would be on guard for any changes in Maddy's demeanor or appearance. I was constantly taking his temperature, praying for no fever. It broke my heart to see my son weak with no energy. It is tough for any parent to watch their child in any kind of pain or discomfort, but for a parent of a child with cancer, it is brutal. I didn't want to pack our bags knowing that we may be admitted to the hospital. I didn't want to have to take Maddox outside in his condition. I didn't want us to spend the day in an exam room. I wanted him to get rest in his own bed. I tormented myself with thoughts of, "Why couldn't he just be a normal kid and get well at home?!" Well, "normal" would not be in our vocabulary for a long time.

Throughout the day, I would do my best to keep Maddox and Danika apart so that Danika wouldn't catch whatever it was that Maddy was fighting. This alone took some effort. Sometimes Maddox would cry from feeling sick, but not know why he wasn't feeling well. I would do my best to comfort and hold him, hoping and praying that whatever it was would pass. One moment, the thermometer would show a borderline mild fever and I would be instantly on alert, then the next moment, it would be normal and I would feel an ounce of relief. It was incredibly frustrating when his temperature fluctuated like this. We would be in limbo-land. I didn't want to jump the gun and send him to clinic in case it resolved itself, but at the same time, I didn't want to misjudge Maddox's condition. In the midst of all this, I had to take care of my little girl who also wanted and needed her mommy. I often felt all alone with no support, fearful of making any wrong decisions. Brad was at work. There was no way he could assess the situation and there was nothing he could do to make it easier. I was the one that was home. I was the one who was experiencing these events unfold. It would have to be my judgment on what to do next -

keep monitoring Maddy's condition or bring him to the clinic.
Brad relied on me to make that decision.

Having to keep this careful watch on my son for hours was
emotionally draining. There were some rare occasions when
Maddox would snap out of it, but in most cases, after hours of
willing it not to be so, Maddy would eventually develop a full
blown fever. Game over. With a heavy heart, I would get Maddox
ready for the clinic. Brad would head home, oblivious of the
emotional roller coaster I went through that led up to him getting
that second call. I again envied Brad that ignorance. The only
consolation for us going to the clinic was that we didn't have to go
to the ER. At the clinic, Maddox would be seen and examined by
doctors, nurses, and staff that knew his medical history and
information. Maddox's blood would be drawn by nurses familiar
with the procedure of accessing his port. If Maddox happened to
be admitted to the hospital, it would be done through the clinic,
which was a much simpler process compared to going through the
ER. Having to pull Maddox out of the comfort of his own home
and pack us up was never easy, but following a fever, going to the
clinic was always the better alternative than going to the ER.

Regardless of whether it happened in the day or in the night, it was
no picnic whenever Maddox got a fever. Throughout the course of
his treatment, my heart sank every time I noticed that Maddy was
not feeling well. It sank even more every time it happened after
5PM. Fevers at night would often require a trip to the ER and that
always meant that Brad and I were in for a very long night.

Chapter Twenty-Seven

Here is how the drill went whenever Maddy got a fever *after* 5PM.
Once I took his temperature to confirm a fever, I would call the
after-hours clinic to let them know what was going on. They
usually told us to go straight to the ER, but many times I would ask
if I could just please, please wait an hour to see if the fever goes
down on its own. As long as there were no other concerning
symptoms, they often granted us this leeway. Since this was after
5PM, Brad was usually home from work so both of us were able to
keep track of Maddox's condition. Having Brad there was a huge
help because I didn't feel so alone. Both of us were there to take
care of our son. It also allowed us to take turns watching over
Danika, while the other focused on Maddox. It was a big comfort
to have someone else there to help monitor the situation and be the
voice of reason. The weight of the responsibility didn't feel so
heavy when the question is, "What should *we* do?" instead of,
"What should *I* do?"

In talking to a couple of the other moms at the clinic, I know there
were some husbands that just completely checked-out, that didn't
want to play a significant role in their child's care. Yes, there were
certainly many fathers that were very supportive, but from what I
heard, there were other fathers that never even went to the clinic. I
think it was because some of them were in denial, but mostly, I
think it was because most of them were scared. Let's face it,
cancer is pretty scary. I was very thankful to have Brad, a husband
and father who always put his family first. It made such a
difference, especially on nights like this. Every time Maddox got a
fever, there I would be, taking his temperature like every five
minutes, willing it to go down. In my desperation to keep Maddox
and us at home, I would continue to take the temperature in one
ear, and if that was still high, I would take it on the other ear,
praying that maybe that other ear would show no fever. I knew I
was postponing the inevitable, but I wanted to do everything and
anything I could to avoid going to the ER. For some reason, I
never trusted the first thermometer reading, especially if it read
high. I would always have Brad take the temperature again after

me, as if by having him do it, the results would be more reliable. Whether or not that made any sense, it didn't matter. It just felt good to have him there to support me no matter how many times I took Maddy's temperature. I thought of the other moms whose husbands were not involved and I admired these women for the incredible courage and strength it must have taken for them to handle all of this on their own. It made me even more grateful that I had a partner through all of this. I know I was upset that Brad wasn't more involved in helping with Maddox's chemo at home, but the truth is, he was there for me and our family in many other ways.

Once the hour was up and Maddox still had a fever, we would have no choice but to reluctantly inform the after-hours clinic that we would be on our way to the ER. I would reluctantly pack a bag of our clothes and toiletries knowing very well that we would probably be admitted to the hospital. Once the bag was packed, I would prepare Maddox for the visit by placing lidocaine over his port. This would numb the area so they could draw Maddy's blood with no pain.

Going to the ER was extremely grueling. Since this pediatric ER did not specialize in children with cancer, there were kids there for all sorts of reasons, from a broken bone to a bad case of the flu. I always had to inform the front desk that Maddox was in treatment so that they could at least place us in a different room to protect Maddy from whatever viruses were floating in the air. Before waiting to go to the exam room, one of the nurses would take Maddox's vitals, which included getting his blood pressure and temperature taken. They would then make him stand to get his height and weight. It would be late and by this time in the evening, Maddox would be very irritable and understandably so. Sometimes he would cry, hating every moment the nurse touched him. There he was, with a fever, having to go through a series of exams when all he probably wanted to do was lie down and rest. I hated that he couldn't be home to do just that.

When it came to the ER, there was a lot of waiting. We waited in the waiting room to be called in to get Maddox's vitals, we waited even longer in the exam room for a doctor to see him, and once Maddox finally got his blood drawn, we did some more waiting to get the results. In the beginning, I often took Maddox to the ER because I knew all of the medication he was taking, and his medical history. Since this was not the clinic, the attending physicians and nurses were not familiar with Maddox's medical history and they did not specialize in the care for cancer patients. Therefore every time we went to the ER, we always had to recite Maddox's medical information. Brad stayed with Danika while I called him with updates. The attending ER physicians would be in communication with one of the pediatric oncology doctors on duty, who would then instruct them on the proper protocol to follow. This protocol mainly involved getting a CBC, Complete Blood Count. Some nights you could tell that the nurse on duty was not familiar with accessing ports. Maddy always seemed to sense this and he would squirm and cry when the nurse would attempt to access him, afraid that they were going to hurt him. I would be holding Maddox against me on my lap to keep him from punching and kicking the nurse, while I watched her basically learn, on the spot, how to access the port. Thankfully, the lidocaine would numb the area so Maddox never really felt any pain. He was more scared that the nurse didn't know what she was doing. Frankly, I was too. Once he was accessed, Maddy's port was typically hooked on to an IV with saline water to keep Maddox hydrated. The IV was also put in place to administer any antibiotics should the doctor order them.

Some nights, we would be at the ER for hours. Maddox would be so tired and cranky until he was too exhausted to do anything but pass out. I would let him lie on the exam room bed and rest as much as he could. They were not very comfortable beds and it was often cold in these rooms. I often laid down with him to keep him warm and to comfort him. Other times, I would just sit quietly in a chair in the dim room just watching him sleep, listening to the faint sounds of the intercom paging this doctor or that person, and listening to the beeps of the blood pressure machines down the hallway. I would just sit there with as much patience as I could muster, waiting for the sound of a knock to let us know whether we could go home.

The rest of our night would be determined by a blood test. Should his white blood counts fall below a certain number, we would be admitted to the hospital. Often, when all was said and done, the counts would not be in our favor. I would then make that call to Brad to let him know that Maddox was being admitted. A lot of nights, it would already be midnight or later when we would yet again have to wait, this time for a hospital bed to be ready. Some nights it would be two or three o'clock in the morning before we got a room. My mind and body would be weary from exhaustion by the time we were escorted to the pediatric wing of the hospital.

Our stay would be at least three days because that's how long it took to get the results back from the blood cultures. Brad would coordinate with his job to allow him to work remotely or to take some time off. That being said, I have to take a moment to mention how incredibly supportive Brad's company was throughout all of this. We were very grateful for the flexibility his job afforded him. Because of that, we were both able to be there for our son. We would take turns with Maddox at the hospital until he was discharged.

In order to assess the cause of Maddox's fever, they had to draw his blood regularly, sometimes every four to six hours at a time. They would examine the blood cultures to determine whether there was any unusual growth. Maddy was usually put on some type of antibiotic as a precautionary measure in case the fever was caused by an infection. They could generally tell by the second day whether there was any growth or change in the cultures. If the blood reports showed no signs of growth after two days, and as long as there were no more fevers, we were generally discharged by the third or fourth day. By that point, whether or not the cause of the fever was discovered, they felt comfortable sending us home. Anytime Maddox was admitted to the hospital for a fever, we knew that we would be there for a minimum of three days. On a very rare occasion, they may have released him after two days. The fevers were often a marker to how long we were going to be at the hospital. If a fever persisted past the second day, blood would continue to be drawn and a new set of cultures would be examined for any growth. This would essentially be the protocol until there were no more fevers. The longer Maddy's fever persisted, the longer our stay would be at the hospital.

Chapter Twenty-Eight

It is difficult to think back to those nights at the ER and the subsequent hospital stays. Those were some physically and emotionally draining times. Brad and I were all too familiar with the routine during those stays. The doctors would come in the early morning to do their rounds. The nurses came every four or six hours during the day and wee hours of the night to take Maddy's vitals. Other nurses would come in at different times to draw Maddy's blood or check on Maddy's IV to refill or reset the drip. I remember too many times at two, three, or four o'clock in the morning when Maddy or I, or sometimes both of us would be rudely awakened by the sharp beep of the monitor letting us know that the IV bag had to be replaced. During these hospital stays, Brad and I knew that rest would be few and far between - for all of us. Sometimes, Maddox was able to sleep right through many of these "interruptions." Other times, he did not. To be honest, I didn't care so much about me. I really just wanted to make sure they didn't disturb Maddox because trying to calm a cranky Maddox often made for a very long and draining night.

One time during an after dinner conversation, Brad's parents made a comment that throughout Maddox's treatment it was "amazing" that he rarely had to be admitted to the hospital. I guess from an outside perspective, it would seem that way, and perhaps compared to some of the other children in treatment, that was the case. Of course we were very thankful for that. However, with all due respect to Brad's parents who I love very much, I just remember sitting there quietly thinking to myself, "Were they serious? It wasn't 'amazing' at all. Did they not realize how often we had to go the hospital?" For Brad and me, Maddox was admitted to the hospital more times than we'd care to remember. For us, each and every hospital stay was one too many.

Knowing what those hospital stays were like, I was fiercely determined to do everything I could to avoid them. What some people didn't understand was, this is why I was so very careful and watchful about not exposing Maddox to any germs. Of all the precautions we took and there were many, one of the toughest for me was that I actually refrained from hugging and kissing my own son. Obviously, I didn't allow such contact if I had the slightest hint of a cold or cough as any parent would. But even when I was perfectly fine, I found myself holding back. Yes, I actually chose to refrain from expressing the most natural and basic instinct of love and affection a mother can show her child. There were so many times that I just ached to hold him close and kiss him, but I didn't. In the back of my mind, I thought if Maddy got sick from me, I would never forgive myself. When I did kiss him, it was always on his head or his arms. I made sure not to kiss him on the mouth or his face. When I did hug him, it was always from behind, with my face turned away from him because I thought that would better protect Maddox from being exposed to any germs. What an awful and unthinkable thing for a mother, who loved her son so much, to feel compelled to do. Having to police myself from showing physical affection to my child hurt me so deeply. While this was not on the long list of safety measures we were instructed to take, I was so petrified of Maddox catching anything that I just didn't do it.

I remember one time when Brad's parents were visiting, they mentioned that one or both of them just got over bronchitis, or a cold, or something like that. I knew they were fine, otherwise we never would have let them come and visit. Well, they barely walked in the door when I remember saying something like, "Just to be safe, no hugs and kisses." Could you imagine telling grandparents not to hug or kiss their grandchildren?! Impossible! It was not the easiest thing to ask of them, but I sure as hell did. They probably thought I was going a tad overboard, but God bless them, they listened. I got grandparents *not* to hug or kiss their grandchildren. Wow. Not one of my finest moments.

Even with Brad, I cringed in fear anytime I saw him kissing Maddy on the mouth or hugging him close. It took everything in me not to stop him. I would not take that affection away from Brad or Maddox. One over-the-top parent was enough. I know that I may have taken my safety precautions one step too far, but the overprotective Mama in me overruled the practical. I was so jealous of Brad's ability to not overthink things. Unlike me, he never let his worries get in the way of his hugs and kisses. Thank God for that. If only I allowed myself the freedom to just let go. Countless times I wished I was able to just simply throw caution to the wind and embrace and hold my son without a care in the world. But the world we lived in was a world where my son was battling cancer. That was a sobering thought. It breaks my heart that I felt compelled to take what were probably unnecessary measures in order to look out for Maddy's well being. In hindsight, I don't think I would have done anything differently. The fact was, our son was getting chemo treatment. That made him very vulnerable. It may not have made sense to anyone but me, but I thought if holding back my hugs and kisses could somehow keep Maddy well, then it was a sacrifice that I had to, and was willing to make. A mother's job is to protect her children and that's exactly what I was determined to do.

Yes, I Purelled and washed Maddox's hands a lot. Yes, I made Brad install a Purell dispenser by the door. Yes, I made the kids change their clothes every time they came home from outside. Yes, I would use a separate sponge when washing the kids' dishes to prevent them from being contaminated. Yes, I made every single person wash their hands and take their shoes off before coming into the apartment. And yes, I even deprived myself of showering my amazing son with the countless hugs and kisses I wanted to give him. I said yes to anything and everything I could do to protect him. If he caught something serious, his body and immune system were not equipped to fight back. As much as humanly possible, I made it my job to make sure Maddox was kept safe. I know there are those that thought I was crazy and way too overprotective. Maybe I was, but you know what, I really didn't give a fuck. I don't think these people realized that I had a very strong motivation for taking all those extra precautions. I knew, KNEW with complete certainty what would be in store for us if Maddox got sick. When most children got a fever, the standard protocol would be to call the pediatrician, give them some Tylenol, and call it a night. When our son got a fever, it almost always meant spending several physically and emotionally exhausting days and nights at the hospital. For Maddox, that would mean a myriad of exams and blood tests. For sweet Danika, that would mean having part-time parents until we brought Maddy home. For Brad and me, that would mean long and draining days vigilantly watching over our son, praying for a quick recovery. If there was something I could do to prevent all of that, you're damn right I would have done it. So, was I a tad overprotective? Probably. Do I apologize for that. Hell NO.

Chapter Twenty-Nine

The Clinic

As part of his treatment, Maddox would attend regular clinic visits for his check-ups and his scheduled procedures, as well as to get chemo through his IV. Among the many toys at the clinic, there was a play kitchen there that Maddox loved so we began referring to the clinic as, "the kitchen." Every time we had an appointment, we would tell Maddox we were going to "the kitchen." Whenever he heard this, he would light up because he knew he was going to a place that had lots of toys and his favorite little kitchenette. Renaming the clinic in child-friendly terms took a lot of the fear away from him because when he heard it, he would not associate it with getting chemo, instead he would associate it with something fun. It was important for us to make our son feel as safe and secure as possible, so for a while, the clinic became known as, "the kitchen."

In the beginning, Brad and I would take Maddox to these appointments together, but since Brad had already taken several weeks off from work during those weeks at the hospital, it was important for him to get back to his regular schedule at work. Eventually, I took Maddox to his clinic visits and Brad took on the responsibility of bringing Maddox to the ER whenever he got a fever at night. At these clinic visits, patients were seen mainly in the mornings, usually on a first come, first serve basis. Sometimes no matter how early we got there, we would still find ourselves at the clinic for hours. The first thing Maddox had to do was get his vitals taken and blood drawn. Thanks to his port, Maddox's blood draw was fairly easy. If there weren't a lot of children scheduled, we were called in right away to get this done. Once his blood was drawn, we had to wait for the CBC's from the lab to come in before any chemo could be ordered and administered. Basically, we could not do anything until we got Maddy's counts. Sometimes the labs came in quickly, and other times we would find ourselves sitting there for hours. I'm sure it would have been more efficient if the lab just handled the pediatric patients, but since it was the lab for the entire hospital, some days they would not get to us for a while.

Once Maddy's CBC's were confirmed to be good, we would have to wait again - this time for the chemo to finally be ordered, mixed, and picked up by the nurses. There were days when things would run very smoothly and we would be in and out of the clinic "quickly" within 2 to 4 hours. In my opinion, those days were few and far between. A lot of times, especially when Maddox was scheduled for a procedure, I knew we'd be spending most of our day at the clinic. Sometimes, Maddy had to get an IV infusion of chemo rather than a simple push through a syringe. These infusions were not as quick as a push. The infusions ranged from taking thirty minutes to several hours. This was especially so whenever Maddy had to get a blood transfusion. It was not the easiest thing to watch whenever my son had to get a blood transfusion because in my mind, it was some stranger's blood going into his body. I would look at that bag of blood, wonder who it belongs to, and pray that it is compatible, good, and healthy blood. Since no one in our immediate family was a match for Maddy's blood type, he had to get it from the hospital's blood bank. That can be a daunting thought, but ultimately, I was incredibly thankful because it would supply and replenish my son with the much needed components or "nutrients" his own blood happened to be lacking at the time. It made me so grateful to all the blood donors.

The days that Maddy had to get a blood transfusion were especially tedious for me. This was way before we owned any I-pad or I-phone so there was very little I could do to entertain myself. There were only so many magazines I could read before they all blended together. By the end of the visit, I would be more exhausted from basically doing nothing. Sometimes just the mere act of waiting around took the most effort. It was definitely a lesson in patience. Thankfully, Maddox never really minded as long as there were toys he enjoyed and of course, a TV or DVD player to watch his favorite shows. We learned early on that those mini DVD players were a hot commodity at the clinic and so, Cathie, Maddox's grandma, kindly bought us one of our own.

That little DVD player would be a godsend during some of those long days at the clinic. Forget the diapers! It was the DVD player that I made sure was always in the diaper bag.

Chapter Thirty

One of these clinic appointments was brutal. Maddox had to get an injection of chemo right into his thigh. This was a very painful injection called, asparaginase. It was given during the Intense Phase of Maddy's treatment. Maddox had gotten this injection once before when we were at the hospital. The first time he got it, Brad was told to hold Maddox close to keep his arms down, while I was instructed to hold Maddy's legs to keep him from kicking. Right away we knew this was going to be unpleasant. That would be an understatement. We listened to our son scream in fear and horrific pain as the nurse gave him this injection. Brad and I experienced our own agony at having to witness our son suffer such pain. As parents all we want is for our children to feel safe and protected. Yet there we were helpless to stop any of it. At least that day, Brad was there with me. At the clinic, it was just me.

Before administering the shot, the nurses showed me how to hold Maddox. Seated in the chair, with Maddox on my lap, facing away from me, I placed my arms over his arms, hugging him close from behind, and I wrapped my legs crisscross around his legs. Then, I braced myself. The nurses knew it was going to hurt. I knew it was going to hurt. Maddy must have sensed this too because whimpering, he started to squirm in an effort to break free from my hold, even before the nurse took out the needle. Maddy was little, but he was very strong. When the needle finally went in, he fought and fought trying to escape. Maddox with tears streaming down his face was *screaming*, "No! No! It hurts! All done! All done!" Holding back my own tears, I squeezed my eyes shut and just held him tighter, as strong as I could, begging for it to be over. When I opened my eyes, I felt drained of all energy. Traumatized and shaken, I just remember thinking, "What is this hell I am in?" I went home feeling depleted and defeated. No parent could ever be strong enough to handle watching their child endure such pain. I certainly wasn't. Later that day, I remember collapsing into Brad's arms finally allowing myself to break down and cry after such an ordeal. Thank God that was the last time Maddox would get that shot.

Have you sometimes ever felt that gripping fear when waking up from a bad dream, thinking it was real, and then a moment later, feeling this overwhelming relief that it was just a dream? For me, it was just the opposite. There were some mornings when I would wake up and for a half of a split second, it would feel just like any other ordinary day. For that brief moment in time, all was well with the world. Then in an instant, this awful sensation would creep up on me. The realization that my son had cancer would fill my chest with such heaviness. For me, there would be no moment of relief. I would lie there letting this sadness settle over my mind and my body. Some days, it would take every effort I had to get up and face the day. For me, the nightmare was very real. Days like that at the clinic made it impossible for me to think otherwise.

Chapter Thirty-One

During these clinic appointments, I would meet some of the other families and we would share our stories. In one of our first clinic visits, there was this one mom I met whose son was being treated for a different kind of cancer. I remember the boy's name was Christian. He was a very handsome little boy. Once in a while, he and Maddy would play together. From what I recall, this mom told me that the treatment for Christian's type of cancer was pretty intense, with Christian having to go through radiation treatment as well as chemo therapy. I remember us talking one day as she very casually and matter-of-factly said that Christian would never be able to have children. What??? Oh my gosh. For a moment, my heart caught in my throat. She was quite calm when she said it. Meanwhile I was stricken with fear and incredible sadness for her and her son. I fought the urge to cry right then and there.

When this mom shared this detail with me about her son, I thought that this had to be because her son was getting radiation. I didn't know for sure whether the radiation had anything to do with her son not being able to have children, but that's how I rationalized it for my own selfish reasons. I convinced myself that since Maddy did not have to do any radiation treatment, then his ability to have babies is safe. That's all there was to it. I was so thankful that Maddox did not have to endure any radiation. I thought of the heartache this mom must have felt for her son when the doctor told her that he wouldn't be able to have kids. I never even thought that could happen. This information was probably found in all of that literature Brad and I were given to read when we had to choose a treatment plan. I made Brad read most of it because so much of the information was too scary for me. I was obviously right.

Such news would be devastating for any parent so I had to believe that this mom somehow found a way to make peace with it. I don't know how I would ever recover from such a blow. As a mother, one of the greatest gifts is to become a grandma and watch your own child know the incredible, immeasurable joy of bringing life into this world. I thought of Maddy and prayed with all of my heart, "Please, oh please God, let Maddy be able to have children. Please God, let Maddox be a daddy one day." Cancer has already taken so much from us, I begged the Lord that it would not take fatherhood away from my son. I know I should have talked to Dr. Del Toro that day about it, but I didn't. I couldn't. I was too afraid to find out the answer. At that point, I was still too emotionally fragile to handle any more than what we already knew. I figured that this is something Dr. Del Toro would have told us and since he didn't, I was content and determined to believe that Maddox's treatment would not effect his ability to have children. It just wouldn't. With that, I pushed those worries far, far away.

Chapter Thirty-Two

The Clinic Walks

At the time, we lived about one and a half miles away from the clinic, which in city-speak is roughly about twenty-five blocks. On a good day, the walk to the clinic was fine. I am a city girl so while a mile and a half may seem like a long walk for some, for me it was very manageable. It certainly made for some good exercise, particularly on those street and avenues where the walk was mainly uphill. During the winter and days when the weather didn't cooperate, many of those walks to the clinic were especially challenging, not just physically, but emotionally as well. Some of the more unpleasant memories I have were the days when it rained. Some days it didn't just drizzle, it poured.

I remember one cold winter day, the rain was down right torrential. Anyone living in NYC would know that trying to catch a cab, in the rain, in rush hour traffic, is basically impossible. Maddox's clinic visits were usually in the mornings so we were right in the thick of rush hour madness. I had Maddox in the stroller with the rain shield over him, and street after street, I desperately tried to hail a cab. I saw many other people on the street corner struggling to do the same and prayed that one of these folks who happened to catch a cab, would take mercy on a mother and her child waiting in the cold rain, and offer us the ride instead. I at least thought that some of the men would have shown us that courtesy. I mean really! Whatever happened to women and children first?! Well that day, with the rain coming down hard, there would be no good Samaritans - or gentlemen for that matter. Fuckers! With a heavy heart and the realization that my efforts would be useless, I resolved to walk.

Every once in a while, with the rain pelting my face, I would glance back with my arm raised hoping upon hope that an available cab would miraculously appear and stop for us. All I saw was cab after cab passing us by. I couldn't really carry an umbrella because I needed my hands free to push the stroller. In the pouring rain, with a flimsy hood my only protection from the elements, I walked as quickly as I could to get to warmth and dry land. The only comfort I had was that Maddox was safely protected from the cold and rain tucked snugly in his warm Bundleme, and under the protection of his stroller's weather shield. Otherwise, there was no way I would have subjected him to any of that. Maddox probably thought the whole thing was a hoot. By the time we arrived at the clinic, I was not only sopping wet on the outside, I was also dripping with sweat on the inside. You have to understand, with Maddox, his diaper bag, and all the other items we had with us, the weight of the stroller gets pretty heavy, especially when I'm practically running. Usually I can walk leisurely to the clinic, but in the rain, I was forced to hustle. On such days, pushing the stroller twenty-five blocks felt more like fifty.

A regular person would have just chalked this incident up as an incredibly huge pain in the ass. Sure, they probably would have complained up and down about their morning commute to friends, as any normal person would. Our circumstances, however, were far from normal. I not only felt defeated when someone besides us caught a cab, but with each passing ride, I found myself getting more and more lost in feelings of despair. The further I walked, the more bitterness built up inside me. It's funny, for lack of a better word, that such an incident that can be fairly described as merely an inconvenience for most, would trigger such a fierce emotional response from me. Sprinting in the rain, with sweat forming down my back, and tears forming in my eyes, I thought, "I wouldn't be getting soaked in the rain if we didn't have to go to the clinic. I wouldn't have to go through any of this if Maddy didn't need chemo. None of this would be happening if my little boy wasn't sick. None of this would be happening if my little boy didn't have cancer." I wanted to scream, "FUCKING CANCER!" With over a mile walk, I had plenty of time to let such thoughts consume me. I was angry, distraught, and exhausted beyond measure. After twenty-five grueling blocks, I would arrive at the clinic that day a physical and emotional wreck.

As much as I'd like to say that was the first and only time that happened. It wasn't. Maddox was in treatment for three and a half years. It should not be surprising that we got rained or snowed on, on more than one occasion on our way to the clinic. In fact, it happened more times than I'd care to remember. Keep in mind that on the day I just described, I had the "luxury" of the option of trying to get a cab. Either Brad was working from home or a babysitter must have been with Danika that day. It's easier to manage getting in a cab with just Maddox and a single stroller. Well that often wasn't the case. More times than not, I had the double stroller. Danika was barely two years old and often had to be carried. Maddox was just three years old. At the time, we had a Phil and Ted stroller. The folding instructions on this model required that you take the back seat out first, making folding the stroller not such an easy task. These days, there are strollers that fold themselves with a simple push of a button. Where was that genius invention when I needed it the most?

With both kids in tow - even if we got a cab - there was no way I could manage putting both Maddox and Danika in the back seat safely without them falling - mind you there are no car seats required in cabs, then getting all of our gear inside, then leaving the kids alone in the cab so that I could remove the back seat, to then get the stroller folded so that I could place it all into the trunk of the cab. Whew! After all that, once we arrived at the clinic, it would probably take us another twenty minutes just to get out of the cab and back into that stroller. A better mom than me probably could have done it, but the logistics of it all were way too daunting. Maybe there would have been a cab driver who would have shown some kindness, but the odds of one them helping me with all of that, especially in torrential rain, were slim to none. With the double stroller, I never even considered getting a cab when it rained. Rather than putting myself and the kids through that, I chose our only other alternative. Walk. Once the kids were tucked in warmly in their stroller and covered up securely with the rain shield, I would brace myself for a long, arduous and very wet walk. With each step, as I made my way through the rain, that stroller would feel heavier and heavier. Even now, I can almost feel the strain on my arms and legs as I gathered the energy to push, or heave it, for a better word, up along some of those uphill blocks.

It wasn't just the rain that deterred us on some of these walks to the clinic. Some days, we had to contend with the snow. In those cases, it wasn't the actual snowfall that was troublesome. It was the freezing cold and un-shoveled sidewalks that would pose the biggest challenges. Anyone that knows me knows that me and the cold don't play well together. Doing my best to ignore the bite of the freezing cold, I remember several walks when I was either navigating the stroller through messy slush, or navigating the stroller and myself, as safely as I could, through slippery ice.

In time I learned to deal with it whenever it rained or snowed on us. I learned to keep my emotions in check. Of course I still got frustrated and aggravated whenever we found ourselves walking in such inclement weather, but the resentment I felt during those first experiences subsided. Oh it was still very much there, but I did my best not to let it overwhelm me. On the rare occasion that Maddox and I did catch a cab, I would not only thank the driver profusely, I would also say a silent prayer of thanks to the good Lord above. Catching a cab not only spared me the long walk, it also saved me from letting my mind wander to some dark places.

Chapter Thirty-Three

It seems that several of these walks to the clinic were just as emotional as some of the clinic visits themselves. Here is another day that I remember quite vividly. I was walking Maddox to the clinic and I soon began to notice lots and lots of children of all ages, and their parents excitedly walking along the streets. For a moment, I was both curious and confused. I was trying to figure out what the heck was going on, when all of a sudden it dawned on me. It was the first day of a new school year! Maddox was still in the Isolation Phase, meaning that except for these clinic visits and our strolls in the park, we were basically just home. One month kind of blended into the next. I guess I was so used to living in our own little "bubble" that I completely forgot what time of year it was. It was September. It should have been Maddox's first day of preschool. Instead he was on his way to get treatment for cancer. Man. Treatment for cancer. It was crazy. I thought about how our lives and how it, in what seemed like a flash, went from the ordinary to the unimaginable. None of it made any sense. It wasn't that long ago that I too was filling out those preschool applications excited for my son's first day of school and the discoveries and friends that he would make. We should have been experiencing this wonderful milestone too.

As these children prepared for school, my son was preparing to get yet another round of chemo. I couldn't help it. My response was immediate. Right there, somewhere between Madison and Fifth, I began to cry. We would pass by several of the school buildings that I was now more aware of, and I would look at all the children out front, happily waiting to go inside. I felt desperate for us to be a part of it all. I would glance at some of the parents and see the looks of eagerness and excitement on their faces. What a stark contrast to what my face must have looked like. Block after block, I let the tears flow willingly. I couldn't care less who saw me. I had so many emotions going through me. I couldn't help but enviously think about my mommy friends who must have been enjoying this special day with their children. I imagined them meeting the teachers and beaming with pride and joy as they took countless photos of their child's first day of school. I thought of them standing watch by the door with the other parents, joined in comradery, worrying about whether or not their child would have any separation anxiety. My worries were *so* very different from theirs. I felt incredibly far removed from all of this. In my mind, I just kept saying, "This isn't fair. This isn't fair." As much as I willed myself to resist it, all I could think of was, "Why us?" It wasn't just about the first day of school anymore. For me, this day truly magnified all the things we were missing out on. I thought about the family vacations we couldn't take, I thought about all the activities Maddox couldn't do, like have play dates or simply go to the playground, I thought about my daughter and how much she sacrificed so that we could take care of her big brother. Yes, I hated, really hated the thought of Maddox missing out on the delights and early wonders of preschool, but as I looked out at all of these people, what hurt the most was that it felt like we were missing out on life itself. All of these thoughts just bombarded my head. As fast as I tried to walk, I could not escape them. I felt sorry for my son, I felt sorry for me, I felt sorry for our whole family. Most of the time, especially when the weather was pleasant, these walks to the clinic were uneventful, but on this particular day, this walk broke my heart.

Chapter Thirty-Four

The Pediatric Hematology and Oncology Clinic had children battling all sorts of life-threatening illnesses. During some of these clinic visits, I would look around at the other children in treatment - some bald, some just starting to lose their hair, some bloated from the steroids, some just pale and weak, and I would feel this deep sorrow. These children were all so brave. Some were just babies.

One morning, Maddy was off playing with some of the toys, and I was waiting for us to be called in for Maddy's chemo. There I was, sitting at one of the tables, when all a sudden, off to the side, I saw a young boy, maybe ten or twelve years old, hunched over, with his mom's arm around him, throwing up into a bag, struggling to let it pass. I figured he must have just had his treatment and was nauseous from the chemo. I quickly turned away feeling deeply sorry for this young boy and his mother. This poor kid should have been off playing baseball with his friends and getting good grades in school, but there he was, getting sick from chemo. I couldn't bear to look at him. It was pretty heartwrenching. I said a silent prayer thanking God that Maddox was spared this side effect. The image of that boy is not one that easily fades. The feelings of sadness and heartbreak at what these kids were going through stay with you for a while. Even arriving home after a day at the clinic, it is difficult to just shake it off. The cumulative effects of going to the clinic month after month and watching these brave young children, including my own son, fight for their lives, deeply effected me.

I don't think Brad or anyone for that matter, with the unlikely exception of Brad's father, Dave, ever completely understood what kind of emotional toll those clinic visits and having to give Maddy chemo every day, took on me. My father-in-law, bless his heart, was the one person who seemed to recognize that I experienced and went through something different, something more. We would have these dinners and as we all reflected on everything that's happened, it would always be Dave that would tell me how amazing I am and how impressed he was by me. In all of these deep family conversations, I honestly was not fishing for any compliments, but it was never lost on me that my father-in-law was the one person who consistently acknowledged that I had to deal with most of the challenges and responsibilities of Maddox's treatment. I have to admit that it felt damn good to know that someone truly appreciated that. I would just sit there quietly and politely smile, when what I really wanted to do was give Dave a big hug and shout, "Thank you!!!" While I never told him how much it meant to me, I always, *always* noticed that *he* noticed. I remember one comment he made to Brad. He said, "At least you get to go to work." That simple statement was worth a thousand words. It said it all for me. My father-in-law got it. In that moment, my wonderful father-in-law was the one person who understood and I loved him so much for it. It was not meant to say that Brad got to go and party all day at work. As I've mentioned, Brad works very hard and I respect him and his work very much. What Dave's comment simply meant was that at least at work, Brad can focus on something else. For me, there was little to no escape from our situation. Of course, without question, Brad and I were equally traumatized and heartbroken that our son was battling cancer. But the fact of the matter was, many of our experiences through it were very, very different. To have someone, *anyone*, acknowledge that, was quite simply, gratifying.

Chapter Thirty-Five

Maintenance

After completing the most intensive phase of his treatment, Maddox was finally in Maintenance. During this phase, in addition to other supportive drugs, Maddy continued to get chemo every day by mouth, and steroids every 4 weeks, but the dosages were lower. He also went to regular clinic visits once a month to get a dose of another chemo called vincristine through his port. On some of these clinic visits, Maddy had to get procedures called lumbar punctures also known as LPs, and Bone Marrow Aspirates. During those procedures, Maddy would also get chemo up his spine. All of this would be our protocol during Maintenance. It may not really sound like it after what I just described, but getting to this phase was a gigantic step for us towards some sense of normalcy. Maddy was in Maintenance! Yes! This phase allowed Maddy and our family to have play dates with other children again, go to the playground, go to restaurants - that was especially awesome, and resume activities that were previously off limits for Maddy's own protection. While this opened up a whole new world for us, there were still many precautions we had to take.

We still had to be careful not to expose Maddox to any germs. As we all know, germs are everywhere, but we did as much as we could to limit his exposure to them. For example, we didn't take any vacations or trips that required any air travel. While this may no longer have been a restriction, getting on a plane where there were too many germs in a confined space was not an option. It just wasn't worth the risk. We did allow ourselves the occasional road trip to visit family and friends, as long as they were a short drive. On all of those trips, I had to pack all of Maddy's chemo and drugs, and all of the gear, masks, and gloves. We also had to be sure to bring all of Maddy's medical records, as well as a letter from the clinic explaining Maddy's chemo protocol just in case he got sick on the trip and had to be admitted to the hospital. As you can imagine, my checklist before getting on the road was not your typical one. When most people travel, their biggest concern is making sure they pack enough clothes. I, on the other hand, had to make sure I didn't forget my son's chemo. It could have easily brought my spirits down and sometimes it did, but eventually, it just became part of the routine, just like packing his toothbrush. Amazing, huh.

To protect his port, Maddy couldn't play any contact sports. We couldn't risk the port getting hit by any balls or sporting equipment. To prevent the port from getting infected, he was also advised not to swim in the ocean or public pool. He was told to avoid certain fruits like raspberries and strawberries. The reason for this is because those fruits have so many nooks and grooves that we would not be able to thoroughly wash the dirt and pesticides off of them. Since apples are heavily sprayed, we always peeled the skins off before serving them to him. We stayed away from any fruits, like grapes and blueberries, that had thin skins. I remember one mom at the clinic told me that she literally soaked grapes in vinegar to sanitize them before serving them to her daughter. Yes, she was that meticulous. Rather than going through all of that, with the exception of peeling the apples, we simply avoided all of those fruits. Maddox sure ate a lot of bananas during that time. It still amazes me how much we did to ensure Maddox's safety and well being. The reality was, while Maddox was in treatment, we had to continue to be very cautious of his exposure. For three and a half years, that would be our way of life. Eventually, it just became part of what he knew, part of how we as a family adapted. Quite simply, Maddox can be a kid again - but under extraordinary circumstances.

Adapt and Overcome. Those are words our family would live by while Maddy was in treatment.

Despite the precautions we had to continue to take, we were so grateful to be in the Maintenance Phase. It was like a breath of fresh air. After so many months of saying, "No, we can't do that" or "No, we can't go there," we were finally able to say a wholehearted, "YES!" to so many wonderful things.

We delighted in trips to the playground and get-togethers with other families, all things that can easily be taken for granted, but not anymore. While we were thrilled to go on play dates again, we had to be careful. Anytime we offered or were asked to go on a play date, we had to make sure that everyone was well. I had to explain that unlike the average kid, Maddox's compromised immune system made him more susceptible to even the slightest of germs. Whenever we got an invitation to someone's house, I had to preface it with, "Please just confirm that no one in the household has a cold, or a cough, or the sniffles." I must admit, at times I was a bit embarrassed to have to say all that. I didn't want to seem rude or offensive, but it was for Maddox's well-being. As I've learned, I had to put his safety above being polite. Of course everyone understood knowing our circumstances, but it still sucked that we couldn't just plan a play date without these "pre-requisites" like any other normal family. Yes, it was an inconvenience, but it was a small price to pay to be able to socialize. It was nice to be able to chat it up with the other mommies again while we watched the kids play, and it was especially wonderful for Maddox and Danika to reunite with their old friends, as well as make new ones. It was a freedom that we held with great appreciation.

Chapter Thirty-Six

In July of 2010, when Maddy turned four years old, we were able to throw him a big birthday party! This was very special to us because it was just a year earlier that we celebrated Maddox's birthday at home, in isolation, with just Brad, Danika, Cathie, and me. With Maddox in Maintenance, we were able to invite many of our family and friends. In addition to the bottle of Purell I placed at the entrance table, there were balloons, lots of presents, a Thomas the Train birthday cake, and lots of smiles all around. So many of the people we love, and who supported us through this journey, were there to share in this special occasion. Everyone knew how much this party meant to us. First and foremost, it was a celebration of Maddox's birthday! On a deeper level, it was also a triumphant celebration of how far we've come. We knew we still had a little bit of a road ahead of us, but having days like this made the journey much more pleasant. The joy on Maddox's face as he played with his friends and opened his presents was everything. For Brad and me, that was truly the best gift of all.

It was during the Maintenance Phase that I was also able to fulfill a special promise. In August of 2011, our family went to Victorian Gardens! For many families, it was probably just another day in the park. For ours, it was a very significant milestone. Maddox was in Maintenance and from there, we were that much closer to the finish line. The first time we saw this amusement park, it was from a safe distance because Maddy was still in the Intense Phase of his treatment. I remember standing there feeling so sorry for us that we couldn't just step right in and be a part of it. We were in such a different place back then. Now, a couple of years later, we were actually there, like a beautiful dream realized. Maddox and Danika went on ride after ride, sporting the biggest smiles on their faces, while Brad and I simply watched, content, and so very grateful. To the casual observer, we were just another family taking their kids to the amusement park. It was a nice feeling to just blend in with all the other families. It felt normal, but I knew that we weren't. Armed with my stash of Purell, I must have sanitized the kids' hands every two seconds. Not normal.

Ultimately, in the grand scheme of things, it was a minor inconvenience. It did not stop us from enjoying every single moment. This little field trip held a lot of meaning because it wasn't that long ago that we couldn't even entertain the thought of taking the kids to that park. It took almost two years to get to Victorian Gardens, but there we were, with Maddox and Danika doing exactly what they should be doing - having fun being kids. It was a happy day for all of us.

Chapter Thirty-Seven

The best part of the Maintenance Phase was that Maddox was given the green light to go to school. Maddox and Danika would both be applying to preschool. I remember the day of Maddox's preschool interview at Merricat's Castle School. Danika had already done her "interview." She was very shy, but allowed the teachers to guide her into the room to play. Maddy's interview was scheduled on a separate day. Basically, this "interview" was just the kids being observed as they played in one of the classrooms.

The first time we applied to this school was before Maddox was diagnosed. Danika was too young so it was just Maddy applying at that time. Well, that first interview was kind of a disaster. There we all were, in the classroom, the children playing, while all of the parents held their breath willing their kids to be on their best behavior, when all of a sudden, Maddox decided that it was the perfect time to have a royal meltdown. I'm not even sure what set him off, but there was no calming him down. I felt all eyes on us and moments later, one of the directors kindly suggested we reschedule the interview for another day. I could literally hear the other parents thinking, "Whew, glad it wasn't my kid." I wanted to disappear. I was completely and utterly mortified! You'd think this happened in front of the Queen Mother for goodness sakes. Looking back, I have to laugh at myself at how seriously I took it. How ridiculous of me. Maddy was just two years old. That's what two year olds do! Well, we ended up getting wait-listed.

We received the school letter in March of 2009 when all the admissions notices were sent, and although we weren't full out rejected, I was devastated at the news. That school was our top choice. I know "devastated" may be a strong word. It's just preschool, but in NYC, applying to a private preschool is like getting into Harvard - and almost just as hard! The preschool process here is unlike any other, and like many Manhattan families, we let ourselves get caught up in it. Who knew at the time that just a few short months later, preschool anywhere would not even be an option. Who knew then that getting into preschool was about to become the very, very, very least of our concerns. Three months later we would get other news that would change everything. Talk about being devastated. That word could not even begin to describe what we felt when Maddox was diagnosed with leukemia. Perspective. Ours would certainly never be the same again. In the blink of an eye, we would get a powerful lesson in recognizing the difference between what is trivial and what truly matters most in this life.

Fast forward to the Maintenance Phase. There we were, once again, interviewing at Merricat's, with all the other parents and children, hopeful and excited. I watched Maddy in the classroom playing and getting along with the other children and I felt so thankful - not because he was behaving, but because we were a part of it. For a very brief moment I wondered what the other parents were thinking when they saw Maddy and his bald head. Then just as quickly as it came, the thought left my mind. It didn't matter. Not one bit. This was a great day for all of us. We didn't know whether our kids would be wait-listed, rejected, or accepted into the school, but just being there was already a huge victory for us.

Everything was different this time around. Unlike the first time, there was no pressure. If the kids didn't get in, we'd be disappointed, but we certainly would not be devastated. I look back at my reaction to getting wait-listed before and I feel so ashamed and foolish. I don't want to take anything away from those parents who place importance on getting their children into the "right" preschool. It's just that after our experience, our view of the world and the bigger picture was forever changed. As much as we loved Merricat's, we knew that Maddox and Danika would be fine in any school, and so would we. The fact that our son could go to school at all, after everything we've been through, was a gift to us.

I can't remember whether it was before or after Maddy's class observation, that I ran into Mimi, one of the school directors in the hallway. Ironically, this was the same director that told us to come

another time after Maddox's meltdown during our first interview.
She remembered me and judging by the look on her face I could
tell that she was confused as to why we were applying again. It
took me a bit off guard. I wasn't expecting to have this
conversation, so I couldn't help but get emotional when I
explained to her what had happened to our son. As my voice broke
trying to hold back the tears, her look of confusion immediately
turned to a look of compassion. She was kind and gracious
towards me and if I hadn't already loved the school, I would have
at that moment.

A few months later, we received both Maddox's and Danika's
acceptance letters. I must confess, I don't know whether my
conversation with Mimi influenced the decision, or whether we
would have gotten accepted regardless of it. Perhaps it was both.
All I knew was that I felt a strong connection to this school. In
fact, out of the five or six preschools we applied to before Maddy
was diagnosed, it was the only private preschool we re-applied to
after getting the okay from Maddy's doctor. If we didn't get in, we
would have been fine sending our kids to a preschool alternative.
But, whatever you call it, intuition or instinct, I knew that we
belonged at Merricat's. I just had a good "feeling" about it. Even
in the early days of researching numerous preschools, both private
and alternatives, I was always drawn to this school. I may not
have known it at the time, but applying to Merricat's would be one
of the best decisions we ever made. It was like God was looking
out for us, leading us to this place knowing that the school and the
people would play a meaningful part not just in our son's journey,
but in mine as well.

Chapter Thirty-Eight

Sometime before starting school, we had the opportunity to sit down with Maddy's teachers one-on-one to discuss some of the precautions that had to be taken while Maddox was in school. On that day, we met Christine, Karen, Lucy, and Praachi. These women were going to be Maddy's very first teachers. Lucy and Praachi, the two TA's, led Maddy to a rug area close by to play, while I sat down with Christine and Karen, the head teachers. I brought an outline with me that I wanted the teachers and the school to have for reference. This is exactly what it read.

Maddox Shepard

<u>*Important Notes for Teachers:*</u>

* Maddox is being treated for Acute Lymphoblastic Leukemia. He is in remission and is doing very well.

* Maddy is on steroids for 5 days every 4 weeks. During this time, he may be more tired than usual. It is also not unusual for him to go to the bathroom more frequently. He may also need to drink more frequently than other students.

* Should any child in his class develop or get exposed to chicken pox, teachers must tell us immediately.

* Maddox has a mediport located under the skin of his upper right chest which is used for receiving chemo. Therefore, he should not participate in any contact sports.

* Maddox should not be exposed to a child that has been given a live shot, including the flu mist. We realize teachers may not often be aware of this, but should they be informed by a parent that his or her child has received a live shot, please let us know so that we

can check with Maddy's Doctor on whether or not to keep him home.

* Maddox receives IV chemo once a month. On those days, he will be out of school.

* Maddox should not play in the grass or handle dirt with his hands. He can play in the grass superficially, but he shouldn't roll around in it.

* He should not handle sand with his hands or play in a sandbox.

* He should not handle plants or soil with his hands.

* Restrictions: No Peanuts, Raspberries, Strawberries, any berries, grapes, and fruit with thin skin. Apples are okay as long as they are peeled.

* As often as possible, please make sure Maddy washes his hands, particularly after recess and before lunch.

Once again, thank you all for your support in protecting Maddy's health. We realize that these are not normal circumstances and we truly appreciate all of your efforts to ensure Maddy's well-being in school.

Gosh, I still remember sitting there in the classroom on those little kiddy tables and chairs going through this laundry list of precautions. I kept thinking to myself, "Wow, this is so much to ask of these teachers." This certainly was not in their job description. The further down on the list I got, the more emotional I got. I felt my eyes well up as I heard myself say, "Maddy can't do this. Maddy shouldn't that. Please be careful of this. Please make sure he does that." It felt like it went on and on. Hearing myself say all of this out loud just made our circumstances all the more real, as if they weren't real enough already. I struggled to maintain some composure. I could tell that Karen and Christine were also trying not to get caught up in the moment. They simply looked at me with warmth and understanding. I knew it was a lot, but when all was said and done, they never let me feel like I was asking too much of them. In fact, it was just the opposite. They didn't give the obligatory nod here and there simply to satisfy me. Instead, they carefully and kindly went through each point in detail with me, being sure to ask questions and make clarifications so that they understood and followed these "notes" to the best of their ability. As we wrapped up the meeting, I looked over at Maddy giddily playing with Lucy and Praachi. I knew right then and there that our son was going to be in very good hands, and that made all the difference in the world.

On Maddox's first day of school, I was so nervous. I know it's the kids that often experience separation anxiety on the first day of school, but in this case, it was me. At home, I had complete control over our environment. While most parents worried about how their child would react after they left the classroom, I had other concerns going through my head. What if Maddy forgets to wash his hands after playing in the yard? What if one of the kids has a cold and coughs on Maddy? What if some kids play ball and accidentally hits Maddy's port? After some moments of panic, I realized that I had to push all of those thoughts and worries aside so that I could enjoy this very special occasion. My son was going to school! I remember putting him in the stroller and before we left, Danika gave her big brother a big kiss. Danika's first day of school was later that week.

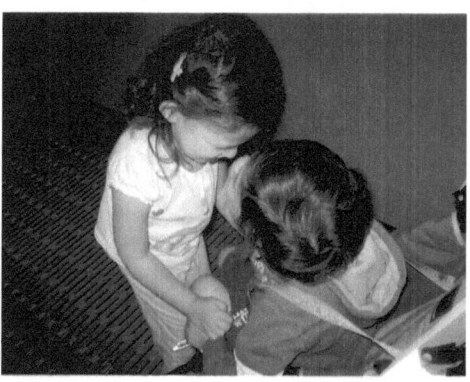

Upon arriving, Maddy showed no signs of anxiety whatsoever. As we walked into the classroom together, I immediately saw one of the TA's greeting the kids on the rug, and I said, "Look Maddy, there's Praachi!" While some of the children clung on to their parents, Maddy walked over and happily plopped himself right next to Praachi. We were allowed to stay for a short bit as the children acclimated themselves to their new surroundings. They sat in a circle with the four teachers who led them in a welcome song. Some children needed more reassurance and had their parents sit with them on the rug, while the rest of us parents observed from the other side of the classroom, all of us with cameras and video recorders on hand, documenting this wonderful milestone.

I watched Maddy singing joyfully and clapping his hands to the songs, perfectly content sitting next to Praachi. He was just loving it. Maddy had no separation issues whatsoever. I felt so proud. Pretty soon, the parents were gradually and subtly escorted out. As I walked out of the classroom, I couldn't help but notice some of the moms crying as they lingered in the hallway not quite ready to let go. I'm sure it was from the thought that their babies were "growing up." I too felt the same emotions, but I did not cry. Maddy was happy. The big smile on his face just warmed my heart all over. I left the classroom filled with hope. I too wore a big smile. I would not shed any tears that day. Finally!

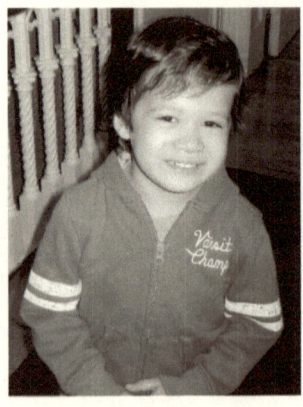

First Day of Preschool!

Sometime that first week of school, as I was waiting to pick up Maddox, Mimi, one of the school's directors, approached me with an idea. She wanted to send a letter to all of the families in the school informing them that a student was undergoing chemo treatment for leukemia. She would use the notes I had given them as a guide and name Maddox as the student. The purpose of the letter was not just to make these families aware, but also mindful of the necessary precautions we had to take to ensure Maddy's well-being in school. Mimi wanted to get my feedback on revealing Maddy's name, as well as my permission on sending the letters out right away. Permission?! I wanted to hug her! Of course she'd have my approval. I didn't even think about doing that. Some people may have thought we should have kept it all private, but armed with this knowledge, perhaps parents would think twice about sending their sick child to school, and instead keep them home, knowing that by doing so they could prevent exposing Maddox to anything harmful. With that said, one of the things I wanted to be clear about in the letter was that we would never make any parent keep their child at home. No matter what, it was certainly not our place to do that. It would be on us to keep Maddox home as we felt necessary. All in all, I thought it was a great idea to have the support of all the families in keeping Maddox as safe as possible. This letter provided a brilliant way to do that.

Once the word was out, the response was incredibly moving. The whole community of faculty, teachers, parents, and students came together to protect this one child, our Maddy. Parents were so proactive in keeping the school informed whenever their child displayed any symptoms of illness. Large or small, they called. Anytime there was even the slightest hint of a student not feeling well, we would immediately get a phone call from the school to let us know. It would then be up to us to decide whether we felt okay sending Maddy to school. Whenever we weren't sure, we would consult Maddy's doctor. Just having the information allowed us to plan accordingly. While we couldn't prevent everything, having this system in place was a huge help to us.

Despite our best efforts, we knew realistically, just like most preschoolers, that Maddy would eventually catch the common cold or some form of it. Preschoolers in general are notorious for being germ carriers so it would have been a tremendous feat had Maddy been able to avoid it all together. The thing is, for Maddy, catching a cold would be anything but simple. If it came with a fever, even a common cold would warrant a trip to the hospital. While this sometimes could not be avoided, all the steps taken to protect Maddy meant so much to us. This school and the families showed us a kindness and love that really moved us.

I remember this one day in particular. Maddy was out of school because he was at the hospital recovering from a fever. He had already been at the hospital for several days. Brad was with Maddox while I went to the school to pick up Danika. I don't remember all the details perfectly, but I must have stopped by Maddox's classroom as well. One of Maddy's teachers asked me how Maddy was doing and as I explained that he was doing okay and recovering, she handed me a small shopping bag. It was a care package for me to give to Maddox at the hospital. I was taken aback by the kind gesture, but I shouldn't have been surprised. That is just the kind of thoughtfulness I had come to know at this school. With tears in my eyes, I thanked her. As I left, my friend Patricia, one of the moms on line to pick up her son, stopped me and asked where Maddox was. I was already emotional at getting the care package so when I told her that Maddy was at the hospital, the tears came rushing back. With tears forming in her eyes too, she hugged me and offered help if I needed it. Patricia was one of the kindest and most considerate parents we met at this school.

When Danika and I arrived home, I looked inside the care package and noticed what looked like a book made of several pages of colorful construction paper kept together by yarn. When I realized what it was, I lost it. All the emotions that were building up throughout the day were let loose. My eyes were blurry from crying as I turned each and every page. It was a card made by all of Maddy's classmates telling him that they missed him and to get better soon. The teachers helped with the writing, but all of the drawings and art work were done by the children. The best part -

each friend signed his or her name as best as their little hands knew how. It is so fitting that the name of the classroom was, "The Friends Room." This thoughtful card truly represented what it meant to be a friend. These children and the teachers could not have found a better way to show that they cared. It was one of the most beautiful things I had ever seen, and I knew that Maddy was going to love it too.

To this day, I am amazed and so very humbled at all of the efforts the school and everyone made to protect Maddy. The fact that they came up with that letter showed us how involved they were with looking out for Maddox's well-being. It demonstrated a level of caring that I'm not sure we would have gotten at any other school. Later, as you read my story, you will know just how far, above and beyond the call of duty, the school and it's directors, Mimi, Linda, and Sheryl, went to support our family.

Like I said, I had a good feeling about this place and I was right.

Chapter Thirty-Nine

Before Maddy was diagnosed with ALL, he was evaluated per the recommendation of his pediatrician, and later approved to get speech, occupational, and physical therapies at home. While he wasn't an extreme case, at this point in his development, it was determined that Maddy could benefit from such services. When it was time to apply to preschool, we had to go through another evaluation through the CPSE, Committees on Preschool Special Education, to determine whether he qualified to continue the program at school. He did qualify, but then the unthinkable happened. We had to stop the services all together because Maddy was just starting the Intense Phase of his treatment. When he was getting these services at home, Maddy became very close to his therapists, especially Martha and Christina. They were coming to our house regularly so we all got to know each other pretty well. Martha and Christina were amazing with Maddy, always so patient and so playful. When they came they always brought an interesting assortment of toys to facilitate their sessions. I genuinely liked these women and I know that Maddy did too - even though at times he didn't want to do the work and just wanted to play. Overall, Maddy enjoyed their visits.

I think I was at the hospital when I called Martha to let her know what was going on with Maddy, and that we had to stop our lessons because of it. In shock by the news, I just remember her crying the whole time while I was on the phone with her. I knew she loved our little boy too. Sometime that week, the doorman at our apartment building gave me a bag of toys that Martha had thoughtfully dropped off for Maddy. One of them was this red barrel filled with monkeys that you connect and hang together. It was one of Maddy's favorite toys to play with and Martha knew that. It was a simple gesture, but it touched us very much.

Because Maddy wasn't able to go to preschool following his diagnosis, Maddox's IEP, Individualized Education Plan, was closed. When Maddox was given the green light to go to school, we were able to reactivate his case file and put an IEP in place at

Merricat's. This program included the speech, occupational, and physical therapies that he was getting before at home. It was a great service that provided Maddy the individual attention to improve all of these skills. In my opinion, it was a great benefit to have these services, particularly the OT and PT, while Maddy was getting chemo. I think it helped maintain and promote his physical strength, and quite possibly, it may have also offset any weakening effects the chemo may have had on his body.

As Maddy prepared to graduate preschool, we attended yet another IEP meeting to discuss his eligibility for the program in Kindergarten. At the recommendation of his preschool teachers and the assessment of his speech, occupational, and physical therapists at Merricat's, it was determined that Maddy would continue these services in Kindergarten. Maddox was placed in an ICT, Integrated Co-Teaching class, which had two teachers - a general education teacher and a special education teacher. This class provided the speech, OT, and PT services within the general education curriculum. To me, it was the best of both worlds. I was very relieved that we were able to get Maddox into this class. Many parents fight for their children to be placed in an ICT class whether or not their child needed extra services simply because it had two teachers. This was a huge advantage in public school, especially in Manhattan, where most classes are over-crowded. With two teachers, all the children would have a better opportunity to get some individual attention. For us, having two teachers was especially important because of all the precautions Maddy had to take in school.

By the time Maddy was getting ready to start Kindergarten, we were feeling very spoiled. Merricat's was pretty special. Maddy would be attending Kindergarten at P.S 158. I must admit, I was nervous wondering what was going to happen in public school. Would they be as nurturing and protective as Merricat's? Would the teachers be as diligent following the precautions Maddy had to take? Would the school be as supportive of our circumstances as Merricat's? These were just some of the concerns I had as Maddox prepared to graduate preschool. I wondered whether public school would be as sensitive to our situation as Merricat's.

Well, something amazing happened at that IEP meeting for Kindergarten. There were several people in attendance at this meeting, which included Karen, one of Maddy's Merricat's teachers, Elizabeth, P.S. 158's school social worker, Adena, P.S. 158's school psychologist, myself, and I think one or two others. We all sat at a round table going through Maddy's education program when Adena tells me that she is recommending that in addition to the related services, that Maddox also be assigned a Healthcare Para-Professional. Adena explained that essentially the HP would be there to shadow Maddox to make sure that he followed all the precautions we had outlined, like making sure he Purelled or washed his hands as often as necessary, that he avoided playing in the grass, that he didn't eat any berries - basically, the HP would be there to look after Maddy's well-being in school. Before she explained it to me, I didn't even know what an HP was, let alone know that we could have requested one. This was the best thing that could have happened. With that simple decision, my worries and concerns were lifted away. To have someone specifically assigned to watch over Maddox in school was a godsend. Once again, here were people that were doing everything they could to support us. Throughout this journey I was constantly amazed at all kindness we encountered along the way.

Sometime during the first couple of weeks of Kindergarten, I had a meeting with Maddy's teachers, Ms. Nicolo and Ms. Diaz, and his HP, Ms. Ramona, to review the notes regarding the precautions Maddy had to take. There I was with that list. Oh, how I prayed for the day when we wouldn't need that damn list anymore. It always got me so emotional. Reading it magnified just how different our lives were compared to the other families in the class - heck, probably the entire school. This meeting was the first time I formally sat down with Ms. Ramona. She was warm, caring, and funny. I knew right away that Maddy would be in good hands with her. She and the teachers were very supportive and understanding. Just like Maddy's preschool teachers, they were careful to go through each point of my outline with me, and by the end of the meeting, I was confident that they too would do their best to look out for my son. I remember one occasion when I chaperoned one of Maddox's field trips. Without knowing I was looking, I often observed Ms. Ramona diligently Purelling Maddy's hand several times throughout the trip. I smiled to myself and thought, yeah, Maddy was going to be just fine.

Chapter Forty

Thinking back on the early months of Maddy's treatment, I made so many mistakes. How could I not. I was not prepared for any of it. There wasn't a class you could take that teaches you how to give chemo to your child or how to care for a child with cancer. I learned as I went. With the chemo at home, through trial and error, I figured out which juices made the medicine taste just a little bit better. I went through orange juice, apple juice, and water until I happened upon a fruit juice that made the medicine taste more tolerable for Maddy. I also learned, albeit the hard way, that pointing the syringe towards his inner cheeks inside his mouth was more effective than pointing it straight. This prevented Maddy from gagging when the medicine was given.

Administering it every day, I became very methodical about preparing the chemo to the point where I could probably whip up a perfectly measured dose in a minute flat, maybe even less. Every afternoon, and twice a day when he was on steroids, I laid out my gloves, my mask, the pills, the syringes, the fruit juice, and the pill crusher on the kitchen counter. I was like one of those people that worked with a conveyor belt - boom, boom, boom, done. So, believe it or not, as the months passed, it got easier. Make no mistake - it was never easy, but it did get easier. This has a lot to do with Maddox. The more he got used to the routine, the more he too learned to adapt. After about a year, Maddox became pleasantly cooperative when it came to taking his medicine and chemo. Sure, he still grimaced at taking it, but it was no longer a battle. That alone was an enormous relief - for both of us! In fact, it even got to the point where he would sometimes remind me, saying, "Mommy, it's time for my medicine." This was really incredible considering that not too long ago, the whole process was quite an ordeal. Now there he was, making sure I didn't forget. This kid is amazing.

At his clinic appointments, Maddox became a model patient, even helping the nurses with holding the syringes and pushing the plunger down as they injected the chemo. As he got a bit older, he showed more interest in what was happening, and so he became very familiar with the routine at the clinic. For a while, in the beginning, Maddy knew the clinic as the "kitchen." We called it that so that Maddy wouldn't be afraid to go. To him, the "kitchen" was a place to play. Eventually as Maddy got older, we felt it was time to call it what it really was, the clinic. While we were comfortable with that, we did not, at this time, explain to Maddox that he had leukemia. We never talked to him about the cancer he was fighting. At four and five years old, we weren't even sure how much of it would make sense to him. It sure as hell didn't make sense to us. All he really knew was that he had to take this special medicine. Brad and I felt it wasn't necessary to elaborate beyond that point. Maddy never asked why he had to go to the clinic and so we never really went into it. I guess Brad and I weren't quite ready to have that conversation with our little boy just yet and so we didn't.

Maddox was still too young to completely grasp why he had to go to the clinic, but at the same time, it also seemed that Maddy was maturing beyond his years. Whenever we told him we were going to the clinic, he knew that it wasn't just a place to play. In time, he knew that that's where we would see the nurses and Dr. Del Toro, and that's where he would get more medicine. Getting his vitals taken, his blood drawn, the exams, the procedures, the chemo - all of it became "normal" to him. Maddy was just a toddler when he was diagnosed. After months of this routine, he probably couldn't remember a time when going to the clinic was not a part of our lives. In fact, it wouldn't surprise me if Maddy thought that all of his friends did the same thing. He was too young to understand that in fact, everything we were doing at the clinic was so far from ordinary. For the three and half years that Maddy was in treatment, that is what he knew. That was his "normal."

Just as Maddy adapted to the routine, eventually, Brad and I settled into our "roles." For the most part, I was in charge of Maddy's chemo and took Maddy to all the clinic appointments, while Brad took him to the hospital ER whenever he got a fever. Brad taking him to the hospital was a huge help because as I've mentioned, going to the ER was often quite grueling. We didn't assign ourselves those responsibilities, saying who would be in charge of what. It's just how it came to be. Brad did his best to go to the clinic whenever Maddy had a procedure, and every once in a while, Brad did help with giving Maddox his medicine, just as I took Maddy to the ER whenever Brad needed a break. Over time, as we learned to manage Maddox's treatment, Brad and I found a balance with what each of us could do to take care of our whole family. I guess you could say that we found our groove.

Brad also felt more comfortable going on business trips, sometimes going for weeks at a time. This probably would not have been possible had it not been for the generosity of Brad's mom and dad. My parents were retired in the Philippines and while my mother offered to fly in, I knew there wasn't much more that she or my dad could do. At their age, it would have been too much for them to make the long trip anyway. To tell you the truth, as much as I loved them, it was more of a help to me that they didn't come. I had enough on my plate. I didn't want or need the added responsibility of having to look after my elderly parents. All I wanted was to focus on my own family.

Thankfully, Brad's mom was there so that I could do just that. Cathie often offered to stay with me to help with the kids when Brad was out of town. I know it probably wasn't always the most convenient thing for her to do, but she did it, and she did it so lovingly and selflessly. She and Dave never let us feel that we were asking too much. With love in their hearts, they just did it. In fact, we never really even had to ask. It wouldn't be long after hearing that Brad had to travel, that Brad's mom would call giving us her flight information to New York. Having Cathie stay with us for days or weeks at a time was a huge help, especially in the beginning when it seemed like Maddy was going to the hospital a lot. I felt better knowing that she would be there to watch over Danika in the event that I had to take Maddy to the hospital. To have that security, not to mention the convenience, was a great comfort to both Brad and me. Brad was able to focus on work and not worry about us miles and miles away knowing that I had help. While Cathie was with us, Dave would be at home in Rochester by himself. I know there were times when they missed each other, but still, they never stopped offering to make the trip.

Because Dave had to work, it was Cathie that often came. Anytime Brad had to travel for business, Cathie was there to lend a hand. In those first early months that she stayed with us, she cooked our meals, helped take care of the kids, and even did our laundry. More than that, she would provide Brad and me with the emotional support that only a mother can give. She was there to listen as we attempted to make sense of it all, she was there to hold us when all we could do was cry, and she was there to be the voice of hope and reason when all we felt was lost and afraid. That is a mother's love. Essentially, she took care of all of us. She was a mom to me when I needed it the most. I can honestly say that I don't know how we would have gotten through those first difficult weeks without her.

In time, and as we settled into the routine, Brad and I gained more and more confidence, and built our strength determined to get through it all. By the time we got to the Maintenance Phase, we had found our stride, and while we no longer needed as much help, we knew that if we did, it was just a phone call away. Dave and Cathie were a tremendous source of support for our family. There are not enough words to express how much we love them for it. Whenever we needed them, they were simply there. They are the definition of unconditional love.

Chapter Forty-One

Early on, we not only found support from our family and friends, but we also connected with a support organization in NYC known as Candlelighters. This organization, led by Barbara Zobian, is dedicated to providing support to families dealing with childhood cancer. I think it was Brad that came across the website on one of our long days during those early weeks at the hospital. As much as we appreciated the support we got from our family and friends, Brad and I knew that being with other families going through similar circumstances made us feel less alone, that in fact, it wasn't just happening to us. It would be those families that would truly understand what we were going through. There is a sense of comradery in that.

Barbara and her amazing team of volunteers would throw these festive events on holidays and throughout the year for the families and especially, the children. Many of them were held at FAO Schwartz, one of the most famous toy stores in the world - what better place to put a smile on children's faces! There was food, lots of treats, toys, and presents - always, lots and lots of presents for the children in treatment, as well as their siblings. Barbara made sure that no one was left out.

I remember being at the first party at FAO Schwartz. The store had roped off the area by that gigantic floor piano. That area and the party room beside it were reserved just for Candlelighters. I watched the pure delight on Maddox's and Danika's faces when the piano lit up with sound as they stepped on those enormous keys. They, along with the other children, went back and forth stomping on those keys, laughing with glee. Afterwards, a real life Toy Soldier entertained them performing "Chopsticks" on the piano. It made these children feel special in the best possible way. With her boundless energy and love for the children, Barbara brought this joy to many of the families, including ours. At these events, the kids were not cancer patients, they were simply kids laughing and playing without a care in the world. These parties were a wonderful way to celebrate these brave children and the siblings who stood beside them.

One of the many wonderful things that Barbara also does for the organization is host the St. Baldrick's Hero Celebration, an event held each year in March. St. Baldrick's is a foundation that raises awareness and funds for childhood cancer research. At these St. Baldrick's events, individuals not only raise funds for the cause, but many of them shave their heads in solidarity with the children who lose their hair as a result of chemo, hence the name, St. Baldrick's. This event also serves to honor and celebrate the children. While the volunteers shave their heads, the kids enjoy food, lots of sweet treats, dancing, games, magic shows, costumes, tattoos, and face painting, many of which are donated by the generosity of the event's sponsors.

Maddox was one of the Honored Children the first time we attended this event in 2010. That year we were just guests. The following year, inspired by all the good the organization does, Brad led a team in raising money for the charity. While I fully supported his efforts, it was Brad that was the driving force behind the fundraising and our participation in these events. This is where Brad really shined. Since getting involved with St. Baldrick's in 2010, Brad has not only reached out to all of our family and friends to raise funds, with the help of his friend Bill, Brad has even coordinated a way to guest bartend at a local bar so that he could donate all of his tips to the foundation. I remember his first gig behind the bar, Brad was getting $20 tips left and right all night long. It was fantastic! Either Brad was really great at pouring drinks, or everyone was being incredibly generous. Ha! I'm pretty sure Brad would agree that it was the latter. Even Brad's boss at the time, Shelly, hopped behind the bar to shell out cocktails. St. Baldrick's flyers and posters were placed throughout the space to encourage the patrons to donate and tip. I have to credit Lisa, Brad's former admin, who tirelessly solicited even more tips by working the room all night long, passing around a tip hat to all of the people. She was amazing! Everyone was amazing. Overall, it was a fun way to raise money for a wonderful charity. So many of our friends and Brad's co-workers came to show their support for our family. It was that same support that allowed Brad to recruit many of these same co-workers and friends to join his team to raise even more money for the cause.

In addition to the fundraising, each year, Brad, his friends, and several members of his team would volunteer to shave their heads at the St. Baldrick's events in honor of the children undergoing chemo. It is quite inspiring to watch, especially when you see women and young kids volunteering to shave their heads. What a simple yet powerful message to these children that they do not stand alone in this fight. At one event, one incredible child, whose hair just grew back after chemo, volunteered to have it shaved. I was moved to tears at such a selfless gesture. It filled my heart with so much admiration and awe, not just for that child, but for all the children battling cancer. The St. Baldrick's Hero Celebration is just that - a celebration of all its heroes. I can't help but get emotional at these events knowing that our story was just one of many in that room. While the mood is festive, we all know the reason we are there. We are joined together for one common goal, and that is to put an end to childhood cancer.

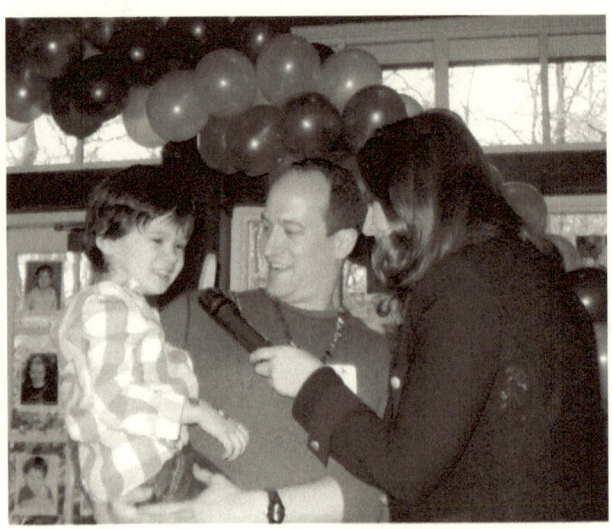

St. Baldrick's Hero Celebration 2011

To date, thanks to the generosity of our family and friends, Brad has raised more than $65,000 for the St. Baldrick's Foundation! What a remarkable accomplishment. When you talk to Brad, he would graciously say that it was due to a team effort from both of us that we reached such an impressive number. While I did my part in supporting him, the truth is, it was all Brad. He led the charge. He deserves all the credit and all the praise. It wasn't just about the money though, Brad really put his heart and soul into raising awareness for childhood cancer research so that one fine day, there will be a cure. He did it for our son and for all the courageous children fighting this cruel disease. I am so proud of my amazing husband for making such a meaningful difference in this crusade.

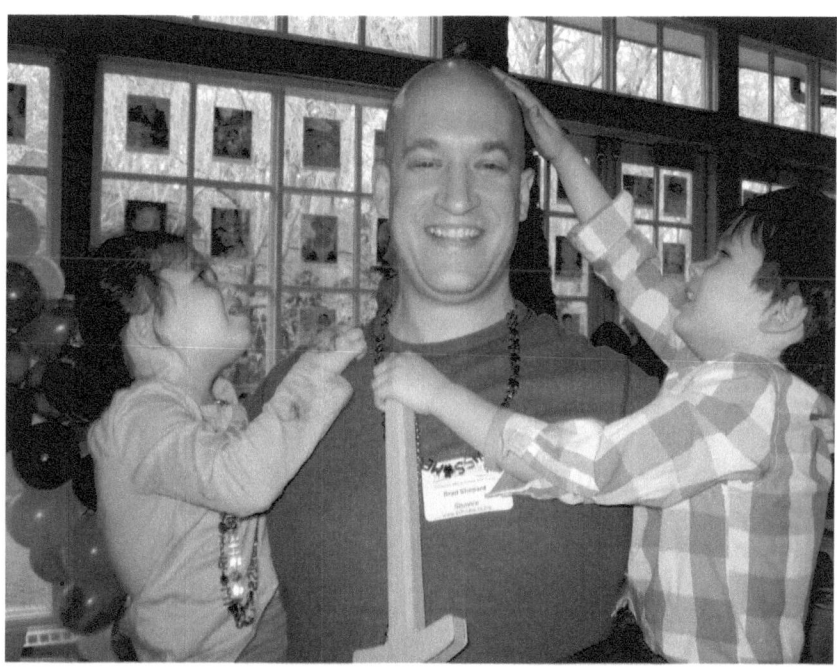

Chapter Forty-Two

Sometime around the second year into Maddox's treatment, two very significant events occurred. The first involved Dr. Del Toro. The second, I'll get to later. The first event happened on one of Maddox's clinic visits. When you walk into the clinic, there is this board on the right wall with pictures on it. One side of the board has photos of the new staff members, and the other side has photos of staff members who were leaving. On this day, I noticed that Dr. Del Toro's photo was on the wrong side. My heart started beating faster. It had to be a mistake. As I checked Maddox in with Jeannette, the receptionist, she confirmed that Dr. Del Toro was indeed leaving the hospital. NOOOOO! There were only two other times that I felt that same urge to yell, "No!" when I found out someone was leaving the department.

While going to this clinic, there were two nurses that we grew very fond of, Nurse Amy and Nurse Megan. When they left the hospital to pursue their careers elsewhere, I was so upset. There are just some people that find their true calling in life and that can definitely be said of Amy and Megan. While most of the clinic staff was wonderful, whenever I saw that Amy or Megan was on duty, I immediately felt a sense of relief. As a parent, you can't put a price on that. They were not just skilled at their jobs, but they also showed a genuine care for Maddy and all of the other children. They always took that extra step. It wasn't just a job to them and we noticed. I knew when they were there that Maddox was going to be in very competent, kind, and caring hands. We had really grown attached to these girls and it was hard to say good-bye to them. Change is not always easy, especially in a place like the clinic where having consistency provides a sense of security. Thankfully, the new nurse, Nurse Rosie became a wonderful addition to the clinic. As we got to know her, she too won us over with her caring ways. While Amy and Megan were hard acts to follow, there were several other nurses at the clinic that we must acknowledge for taking great care of Maddox. There was Chrissy and Tanisha, Lori and Mary Louise, all of whom became part of this journey with us, and we are grateful to all of them.

Once Amy and Megan left, I became more mindful of that board, afraid of who might be leaving next. I would half want to, half not want to glance at it every time we walked in the door, holding my breath, dreading the thought that we would ever see Dr. Del Toro's picture where it wasn't supposed to be. While we had several favorites at the clinic, he was the one person's face we never ever wanted to see on that board. I never thought the day would come, but there it was, staring right at me. Dr. Del Toro was leaving. Yes, there were other fine pediatric oncologists at the clinic like Dr. Wistinghausen who we liked very much, but Dr. Del Toro was our guy. Immediately, my heart sank. When Amy and Megan left, I was incredibly sad. But this was Dr. Del Toro, our fearless leader. I was more than sad. I was heart-broken. What were we going to do??? He was the reason we were there. When you spend so much time in a place, you start to form relationships. We certainly formed a great bond with Dr. Del Toro. In many ways, he became a part of our family. He'd been there with us from the very beginning and we trusted him so completely with Maddy's care. Whether we liked it or not, he always gave it to us straight - the good, the bad, and sometimes even the ugly. We respected him tremendously for that. While this scared us at times, with Dr. Del Toro, we always knew what we were dealing with and that gave us power. Our confidence in him gave us strength when we didn't have any. Yes, there were other competent doctors at the clinic, but Maddox had come to love Dr. Del Toro, and so did we.

When we finally saw him that day, he told us that he had accepted a position as the head of a hospital in Brooklyn, and that he would be leaving in a couple of months. That was a bit of a relief. At least we still had him for another couple of months. I, of course congratulated him and told him had the hospital been anywhere else in Manhattan, that we would have followed him. Going to Brooklyn for Maddy's clinic appointments would just not have been convenient for us. As we talked, I could tell that he was torn. I knew he had gotten close to many of the families here including ours. While we were happy for Dr. Del Toro's exciting opportunity, it was not going to be easy letting him go.

Later that day, I gave Brad the news. He too was shocked and saddened to hear that Dr. Del Toro was leaving. When we finally let it sink in, we thought that it may be a good time for us to make a change as well. For mere logistical reasons, we thought about transferring Maddox to the Memorial Sloan Kettering Cancer Center. By that time we had moved to a larger apartment which happened to be just a half a mile away from Sloan Kettering. This would make Maddy's clinic visits so much more convenient to get to, compared to being almost two miles away from our current clinic at Mount Sinai. For that reason, and of course for the fact that Sloan Kettering is a leader in cancer treatment, it was kind of a no-brainer to make the switch.

Many people wondered why we didn't go to Sloan from the very beginning considering it is a well renowned cancer treatment facility around the world. There were two reasons. The first: When Maddy was diagnosed, we couldn't think about hopping him around from facility to facility for second opinions. We, especially Maddox, had been through enough. We weren't about to put him through another series of tests at another place. All we could focus on was getting him well as quickly as possible. The second: Dr. Del Toro. He gave us the reason to stay at Mount Sinai. Mount Sinai is also a very respectable and excellent hospital, but with Dr. Del Toro leaving, it felt right to make the move.

Before we made any decisions, Brad and I decided to consult with Dr. Del Toro. At Maddox's next clinic visit, we sat down with Dr. Del Toro and told him what we were thinking. On the one hand, Sloan Kettering is an easier commute and a very well respected and highly acclaimed cancer treatment center. On the other hand, Maddy had only another year and a half left of treatment. We wondered whether it was okay to make such a change so close to him being done with his treatment. After all, we were already settled at Mount Sinai and familiar with the routine. We wondered how different things would be at Sloan. We really didn't know much about it except for the fact that it is highly regarded. We talked about all of this and our concerns with Dr. Del Toro, looking for some guidance. Without so much as a second thought, he simply told us that it was a good idea. He went on to say that maybe we won't like it there, or maybe we would have felt that Maddy should have been there from the get go. The bottom line was, he encouraged the transfer. Because Maddy was already in the Maintenance Phase, Dr. Del Toro was confident we would make a smooth transition to Sloan Kettering.

We inquired whether there was anyone there that he could refer us to and he gave us the name of the Director of Pediatric Oncology, Dr. Peter Steinherz. Dr. Del Toro told us that Dr. Steinherz was one of the doctors who trained him. Well, enough said. Sold! We didn't even need to take the tour of facilities. As soon as we heard that, all of our reservations went away. With Dr. Del Toro's blessing and full support, we decided to transfer Maddox to Sloan Kettering. It would be one of the best decisions we ever made.

Chapter Forty-Three

On Dr. Del Toro's last day, the clinic threw him a surprise going away party. A few days before the party, Brad and I took the kids to this arts and crafts place to make a present for Dr. Del Toro. It was one of those places where the kids get to pick a figure and paint it. In this wide selection of figures, I found something that looked like a lizard made of wood. It's tail moved and everything. It was the perfect choice as it held a special meaning for us, and perhaps it would too, for Dr. Del Toro. When Maddy was at the hospital and at almost every clinic visit, Dr. Del Toro would give Maddy these rubbery things that when he threw it on the wall, it would stick. They were almost always in the shape of some kind of lizard. Brad, Maddox, Danika, and I, all took turns painting different sections of the figure and on it I wrote, "Love, the Shepard Family." I would have written more, thanking him and telling him how much we were going to miss him, but the figure wasn't very big! All in all, I thought it was a fitting gift for someone who meant so very much to us.

The day of the party was very bittersweet. There were so many families and staff members wanting to congratulate Dr. Del Toro, but also wishing he wasn't leaving. It's amazing that one person can have such an effect on so many people. Brad couldn't go because of work so I brought the kids to the party. It was held at the Child Life Center of the hospital. I remember sitting at one of the tables with the kids when Dr. Del Toro emerges from hallway, totally unsuspecting of what was waiting for him. We all yelled, "Surprise!" In shock, he took one look at all of us and immediately tears formed in his eyes. I could see him get emotional at the sight of all his little patients, their families, and his colleagues, all of whom came to wish him well that day.

It's hard to imagine that the first time I met Dr. Del Toro, my first impression of him was that he was cold and impersonal. I realize now that in order to be professional, he probably had to shield himself from getting too emotional with the families. Otherwise, he couldn't do his job. It makes me understand even more why he was all business that very first time I met him. Well, I have gotten to know him since our first meeting, and Dr. Del Toro has proven himself to be kind, caring, and compassionate.

Judging by the look on his face as he looked around, Dr. Del Toro was truly moved by the display of affection. There was so much love and gratitude for him in that room, how could he not be overwhelmed by it. There was only one other time that I ever saw Dr. Del Toro get emotional. It was the day that he told Brad and me that Maddy had leukemia. God, that must be a hard job. I can't even imagine what kind of toll that must take on him to be the one to deliver parents that devastating news. I guess that's why he sometimes came off as this aloof, no nonsense doctor. At some point, he probably had to numb himself to survive it and do his job. However, on the day that Dr. Del Toro gave Brad and I the news about our son, he was certainly not numb. At the sight and sound of Brad and I falling apart, I remember looking at Dr. Del Toro's face and seeing the rims of his eyes get red. As professional as he was, he was also human. His eyes began to water, and while he never lost his composure, or allowed any of those tears to fall, it was quite obvious to me that giving us this news deeply affected him too.

At the party, everyone got to witness a tender side of Dr. Del Toro. I think it surprised many people. At perhaps 6'5 or taller, this often serious man is quite imposing, but there, right in front of all of us, he became a big softy. I wanted Maddy to go run up and hug him, but I was caught up in the moment. Now I was crying! As Dr. Del Toro worked the room, there were many hugs shared and presents given. When it was our turn, I had Maddy hand him our special present and we all exchanged hugs with this man who had been such an important part of our lives. He didn't open any of his presents at the party, but I'd like to think that our beautifully decorated lizard is sitting somewhere displayed nicely on a shelf, or on his new desk, reminding him of a family that grew to love and respect him very much.

Once Dr. Del Toro said hello to everyone, we all gathered in one of the rooms where there was a projector screen and rows of chairs. I had the kids sit on the chairs. I stood along the wall with many others as Betty, the Division Manager of the Pediatric Oncology Clinic delivered a beautiful speech in honor of Dr. Del Toro. She was doing a great job up until the very end of her speech when she got choked up and started to cry. Later she told me that it was when she looked at me with tears in my eyes that she too let her emotions get the best of her. She jokingly told me that it was my fault that she lost it. It didn't matter as there were many of us that got swept up in the moment. We all shared in the sentiment of her speech. Several other colleagues spoke, some with funny stories, but most expressing how much they admired and respected Dr. Del Toro. I was amused watching Maddox and Danika sitting there with their cute little hands clapping after each speech. They had no idea what was being said, but with huge smiles, they clapped along with the crowd. It was kind of hilarious and adorable.

After the speeches, we watched a video commemorating Dr. Del Toro's time at Mount Sinai. There were many photos of him at work and him with the staff, but the most touching photos were of those with him and the children. For Dr. Del Toro, it was all about the children. I remember Brad and I asking him one time whether he had any children of his own. He replied that he did not, to which I said to him that the kids at the clinic were his children. He smiled and said, "Yes, they are." Dr. Del Toro dedicated himself to these kids and because of that, he earned everyone's love, respect, and admiration. This party, surrounded by all of the children, the families, his co-workers, and friends, was a wonderful way to send him off.

Chapter Forty-Four

Pretty soon, it was our last clinic visit at Mount Sinai. Strangely, I don't have many memories from that day. We definitely did not make a big deal about leaving so I think only a handful of the staff knew. That's kind of how I wanted it as I really preferred not to have the attention. I never made a formal announcement, so I think those that did know, just found out through the grapevine. I'm sure Dr. Del Toro also informed certain key people, like Rosie, so that we could get the ball rolling on the transfer. A part of me got the sense that some of the staff may have been hurt that we chose to go somewhere else. I do remember Sara, the Child Life coordinator, and Julia, the social worker, telling me how they wish we stayed there to have Maddy finish his treatment, and that they would miss us. Later in confidence, Julia told me that she understood why we were leaving and even talked about how wonderful it was going to be at Sloan. As we prepared to go, Nurse Rosie wished us well and said that all of Maddy's medical records and information were already sent to Sloan Kettering.

We spent almost two long years going to this clinic for Maddy's treatment. It was a part of our lives for such a long time that you'd think I would have been more emotional that day, but I wasn't. While I was very thankful for the people and the care that Maddy got there, I knew it was the right time to make a change. With Dr. Del Toro gone, it certainly made it a lot easier. So with very little fuss, I just vaguely remember thanking everyone as we quietly left this clinic for the last time.

A month later, Maddy and I got ready for his first clinic visit at Sloan Kettering. The walk to Sloan was so pleasant, just an easy straight shot down York Avenue. I didn't have to worry about finding a cab or walking a gazillion blocks. There were no steep hills or never-ending avenues to cross. I just simply walked out my building and strolled Maddy a few short blocks away. That reason alone was worth the transfer. The day would only get better.

In a breeze, Maddy and I arrived at the outpatient Pediatric Day Hospital at Sloan Kettering, and as the elevator doors opened on the 9th Floor, I knew that we had made the right decision. The pediatric clinic was so clean, and modern, and beautiful. It was also very large, probably taking up the entire floor. As we finished checking in, I looked around in wonder. My jaw literally dropped at the sight of it all and it's quite possible that I walked through the place with my mouth open in awe the whole time. There was a soothing aquarium off to the side of the front desk with all sorts of colorful fish. Behind it was a very spacious waiting area with chairs and tables, and some computers, and then there was the playroom. Wow. It was magnificent. Maddox could hardly contain himself he was so excited to get in there. When we opened the doors to the play area, we saw in the corner, a huge playhouse with pint size furniture, and right across from the playhouse, there was a real life kitchen. All around the room there were shelves of board games, shelves of books upon books, all the arts and craft tools you could think of, a large flat screen TV, video games, and countless, and I mean countless toys for kids of all ages. It was like Santa himself delivered every imaginable toy to that clinic. If that wasn't enough, low and behold, we spotted a Thomas the Train table, complete with train tracks and trains. Like a moth to a flame, Maddy went straight for that table. He was like a kid in a candy store! I sat and watched him play happily with his favorite tank engine. I looked around at this amazing facility and for the first time, I thought, "We could have had all this?!" Sure, the play area was nice at Mount Sinai, but this - this took play rooms to a whole other level. This was the mac daddy of playrooms.

It wasn't long before a gentleman approached us and introduced himself as Dr. Gary Mason. He was a Pediatric Fellow that worked alongside Dr. Steinherz. I liked him immediately and so did Maddy. "Dr. Gary," as he would be called by Maddy and us, would be our point person at the clinic. After our introductions, Dr. Gary gave us a formal tour of the clinic before getting Maddy ready for his chemo. I thought I had seen it all already, but as we walked through the halls, Dr. Gary showed us just how huge the place really was. There was a separate room, called the IV Room, where the children got their blood drawn and where chemo was administered. Then there was a whole other area separate from the IV room, where chemo was also given, along with other medication. This larger area was broken up into sections separated by curtains for privacy, and each section had it's own cushy chairs. This area was most likely used for chemo that took longer to infuse. It was like a mini clinic within a clinic. Then there was a private room dedicated to offices, as well as exam rooms. It was quite obvious that Sloan Kettering gets lots of donations and funding. The facilities were incredibly impressive. The clinic at Mount Sinai was quite modest in comparison, with just a handful of exam rooms, and a waiting area that served as the playroom, as well as where the kids sometimes got their chemo. The two were so radically different that I don't think it would be fair to even make these comparisons, but how could I not? The differences were so obvious.

Eventually, Dr. Gary dropped us off at the IV room to have Maddox's blood drawn. Within a few minutes, it was done, and then Dr. Gary escorted us to his office/exam room to go over Maddy's paperwork, as well as to give Maddy a check-up. It couldn't have been more that five or ten minutes after getting into his office that he looked at the computer and said, "Maddy's CBC's look good." I was like, "Wait, what? The labs are in already?!" Wow. I mean we literally just left the IV Room. You have to understand, at the Mount Sinai clinic, we sometimes had to wait hours just for the CBC's to come in. Now, there it was - just moments after getting his blood drawn! I was simply amazed. While we were in the room, Dr. Steinherz came and introduced himself to us. He was a very nice older gentleman, not as imposing as Dr. Del Toro, but still, he held himself with a lot of authority. I liked him. While Dr. Steinherz was in charge of Maddy's treatment, it was Dr. Gary that would supervise it all, and so it would be Dr. Gary that we would ultimately form a closer relationship with at the Sloan Kettering.

Once Maddy's check-up was done, we went back to the play room to wait to get Maddy's vincristine. This was one of the chemo drugs that Maddy got once a month at the clinic. Once again, we barely settled ourselves back in the playroom before we heard

Maddy's name called out telling us they were ready for us. We went back in the IV room, got the quick push of vincristine, said our thank you's, and ba da bing, ba da boom, it was done. A few minutes later, Dr. Gary gave me the chemo calendar for the month and scheduled Maddox's next appointment. Then we were out the door. The whole appointment was finished in under 2 hours. Usually that's how long it would take just to get the CBC reports. We would soon find out that even the LP procedures and Bone Marrow Aspirates were done with the same quick efficiency. Man! This place was a well oiled machine like no other. Granted there were some occasions when we would be at the clinic longer than usual, but those times were pretty rare. Most of the time, Maddy was finished just in time to get to school before lunch. It was quite a wonderful and welcome change.

Chapter Forty-Five

During Maddox's treatment at Sloan, he was admitted to the hospital only once. Maddy had gotten a fever and so we had to bring him to the ER. The hospital at Sloan Kettering was also quite a different experience from what we experienced at Mount Sinai. At Sloan, because they specialized only in cancer patients, Maddox was seen very quickly at the ER and given a room within a matter of moments of determining that his CBC's required hospital admittance. Mount Sinai was a huge hospital with many different departments. As I mentioned before, the pediatric ER there did not differentiate between a cancer patient and a child that was there for say, a broken arm. Because of that, getting through that ER was a much longer process. Getting admitted through the Sloan Kettering ER was seamless. Once again, I was blown away by the efficiency.

The inpatient room we had at the Pediatric Day Hospital was just beautiful. Our room looked fresh and clean, updated and modern. With all due respect to Mount Sinai, it felt like we went from staying at your local average hotel, to staying at The Four Seasons. The only thing that didn't change was the comfort of those pull-out chair beds. I think no matter how fancy the facility, those chairs that converted into beds will never be comfortable. Other than that, the room was really quite nice. Even the food deserves some mention. It was not your typical mass produced hospital food. We actually got menus for breakfast, lunch, and dinner. Each meal included a variety of options, from meat to fish, and there was always a sweet selection of desserts! We were there for about three days and every meal was delicious. Brad and I were flabbergasted - in a good way! I couldn't help but remember all of those countless stays at Mount Sinai Hospital and think once again, "We could have had this instead?!" I guess hindsight really is everything. I remembered all of those exhausting nights at the Mount Sinai ER waiting for hours to get a room. It made me think about how our ER visits and hospital stays would have been so much less stressful had we gone to Sloan from the beginning. The whole process just felt simpler, easier. I knew Brad was thinking the same thing. Being admitted to the hospital was never pleasant, but Sloan Kettering sure made it as pleasant as it could be. As I mentioned, during the course of Maddox's treatment at Sloan Kettering, that was the only time he was ever admitted and that was just fine by us - no matter how "swanky" the hospital.

Chapter Forty-Six

While I have made several comparisons in favor of Sloan Kettering, when all is said and done, I don't think Brad and I have any regrets about getting Maddox's treatment at Mount Sinai. It was the right decision for us at the time. That is largely because of Dr. Del Toro. We were confident in the care Maddox was getting there because of him. For the first two years of Maddox's treatment, Maddox was in very good hands at Mount Sinai.

Another thing to note is that Sloan Kettering is a "center." Its sole purpose is devoted to cancer research and treatment. The Division of Pediatric Hematology and Oncology at Mount Sinai was a "department" within a massive hospital filled with various other departments, from Cardiology to Obstetrics. The Division of Pediatric Hematology and Oncology at Mount Sinai was very modest compared to the grand facilities of the Memorial Sloan Kettering Cancer Center. I have to say that it is because of its "modesty," that the clinic at Mount Sinai felt more intimate. It wasn't just because we were there for two years that we knew all of the regular nurse's and staff member's names, and knew all of the Child Life faculty, but it was because the clinic was such a small department, that we were able to form relationships with everyone. I think that is one of the nicest things we can take away from having gone to Mount Sinai. Once we transferred to Sloan, it was a whole other world. The place was huge with perhaps five times the number of faculty. We probably got to know only a handful of the staff. The nurses were all wonderful and very friendly, but I couldn't tell you any of their names. I guess had we sent Maddy there for treatment from the beginning, it would have been different, but we were coming in towards the completion of Maddy's treatment. I'm sure we would have formed closer connections at Sloan had Maddy been there from the start. A bond that we did form was with Dr. Gary. He was wonderful with Maddox and with us. He easily earned our trust. Like Dr. Del Toro, I knew Maddox was in good hands with Dr Gary, and just like Dr. Del Toro, he too found a place in our hearts.

As different as they were, Sloan Kettering and Mount Sinai both provided Maddox with the highest level of care, and we are incredibly thankful for that. I can't change the decisions that we made. All I can do is trust that we were where we needed to be, when we needed to be there.

Chapter Forty-Seven

Earlier I mentioned that there were two significant events that occurred sometime around the second year of Maddox's treatment. The first was Dr. Del Toro leaving Mount Sinai, which led us to transferring Maddox to Sloan Kettering.

The second event was a shocking discovery I made that none of us saw coming.

Chapter Forty-Eight

My Journey

It was Breast Cancer Awareness Month, October 2011. While there were many ads and commercials publicizing the cause, unbelievably, I never thought to do a self-breast exam. I was aware, but I wasn't concerned enough to perform one. Even after a close friend of mine confided in me that she was diagnosed breast cancer in April of that year, it was not on my radar that it could happen to me.

I had been following and watching the reality program, "Giuliana and Bill." On the show, Giuliana Rancic and her husband were trying to have a baby through IVF. At the time, after flip flopping for several months, Brad and I decided that we would like try to have another baby. On Monday, October 17, 2011, Giuliana announced that she was diagnosed with breast cancer. She said that it was her doctor that made her get a mammogram because he would not move forward with IVF until she got one. I was watching her on the *Today* show and I thought, "Well, Brad and I are trying to have a baby too, maybe I should do a self-breast exam." It wasn't all the advertising on TV for Breast Cancer Awareness Month, but that interview with Giuliana Rancic that made me do a self-breast exam that very night. I have never met this woman, but she probably saved my life.

This is my story.

That night, I was in the shower doing a self-breast exam, and to my utter disbelief, I felt a lump in my left breast. I was stunned. I stood in the shower for several minutes just letting the water pour over me. When I got the nerve back, I felt it again and again to make sure that I didn't make a mistake. I didn't. The lump was very much there. I couldn't believe that I had never felt it before that day. Brad was out of town on business so I was alone with this shocking discovery. I was scared, but a part of me felt emotionally removed, like I didn't want to feel anything. Perhaps it was my experience dealing with my son's leukemia and going through all of that heartache when he was diagnosed, that either strengthened me or more likely, just left me too emotionally drained to be afraid of what was going on with me. I was also in a bit of denial that this could happen, especially after everything my family has already been through with my son. Well, no amount of denial was going to make that lump go away.

After getting out of the shower, I researched and scoured the internet for information on causes for lumps in the breast and found many articles that stated that most are benign. I didn't, I couldn't focus on any of the ones that reported the opposite. I went to bed that night, semi-confident that this was not breast cancer. It just couldn't be. The next morning, I immediately made an appointment to get a mammogram. I was able to schedule one for that Friday. It was the soonest appointment that I could get.

I went in for my mammogram on Friday, October 21, 2011. The findings showed that the lump was suspicious enough to warrant a biopsy. The radiologist even showed me the images of my left breast from the mammogram. He pointed to the lump and I remember that he said something like, the "shape" of lump just did not look right. Anyway, whatever it was, it was enough to cause him concern. They weren't able to schedule the biopsy that day and it happened to be a Friday, so they scheduled it for the following Monday. I thought, "Great, I have the whole weekend to sit on this information, or better yet, lack of information." Even then, I kept my emotions in check.

Brad got home that evening from his business trip and I told him that I felt a lump in my left breast and that I was scheduled for a biopsy. He was concerned, but like me, he did not go into panic mode. He told me everything is going to be okay and that my "girls" were fine. I guess we were both under the assumption that lightening couldn't possibly strike twice.

That following Monday, I got the biopsy. It was fairly quick with just a little discomfort. They said that they would call when the results were ready and off I went with a quiet prayer. As much as I willed it not to be cancer, it was at that point that I kind of knew what I couldn't quite yet say out loud. You know when you just have a feeling about something, well I had that feeling about this. My instincts were telling me that this was not good. Of course, I still clung on to some hope, but I knew.

On the afternoon of October 25th, I got the call. The radiologist said, "The lump is malignant. It is breast cancer." I wasn't surprised. In that brief moment, I wasn't sad or even scared. I was more amazed that I didn't break down. When you hear stories about other women, they tell you about how they break down when they get the news. I was remarkably calm. Like I said, I was either made strong having gone through my son's experience, or I had no emotion left to give for myself. The radiologist explained the next steps and gave me several referrals for breast surgeons to get the lump removed. I felt like a weary, wounded soldier preparing for yet another battle. Here we go - again. WTF.

I told my husband that night when he got home from work that I had breast cancer. He couldn't believe it at first, and even said, "Are you sure?" Yup, I was sure. Being a very supportive and loving husband, he said yet again, "Everything is going to be okay." I mean really, how many fucking times did we have to say that?! Talk about a broken record. Enough is enough! He seemed to take it pretty well and for the most part, was also relatively calm about the whole thing. Perhaps it was him being strong for me or maybe he too had been all cried out from everything we've already been through. Is it possibly that Brad and I somehow found a way to stop or ignore the pain? The answer, as we would soon find out, was no.

We told his parents a few days later. Brad was on the phone with them and after the usual small talk, Brad said we had something important to tell them. He simply said, "Geri has breast cancer." As I listened to him say it, I heard his voice break holding back the tears and it was then that I knew he wasn't that "calm" about it at all. He was devastated by this and probably scared. Could you imagine - first his son, and now his wife was battling cancer. Seriously, What The Fuck?!!! It broke my heart. There we were again, reeling from the hard blow of another sucker punch. It wasn't fair. It was mind-boggling that both my son and I had cancer at the same time. Could the world be this cruel, or are we being punished for some reason? All of these agonizing thoughts went through my head. Over and over again I thought to myself, "What did we do? What did we do? Did we do something in this life to deserve this?" This was the first show of emotion we displayed since we got my diagnosis. My God, how much more of this could we handle??? I didn't cry. I just sat there dumbfounded, feeling empty and drained. With Maddy in Maintenance, we were finally settling into some peaceful territory. Now, there we were, bracing ourselves for another battle. This time, it would be my fight. After telling his parents, we allowed a moment, or two, or three to feel sorry for ourselves. Then, just as we did with our son, we picked ourselves up and resolved to do whatever we had to do to get through this. Never quit. Never surrender. That was that.

Chapter Forty-Nine

After getting this life-threatening diagnosis, I often found myself reflecting on how I was living my life. For several months prior to being diagnosed, I was letting so many of my irrational fears influence the way I was living my life, so much so that I wasn't truly appreciating everything I have. I was letting superstition control many of my actions. I was purposefully avoiding certain things or making decisions based on those notions, thinking that by doing so, I could somehow protect my family and me from any further harm. These superstitions that I adhered to were not based on any logical thought, they were based on pure fear. I was living my life watching and overthinking every move that I made. I guided myself based on these fears because I didn't want any more bad things to happen. I know it doesn't make any sense. In my head, I knew I shouldn't fear things that I can't control, but after everything we've been through with Maddox, it felt like I was scared all the time. In my desperation to try to control everything to keep us free from harm, I allowed myself instead to be a slave to my fears. I was living in what seemed like constant vigilance. It was mentally exhausting. Yet, despite all of these efforts, it still felt like I was just waiting for the other shoe to fall.

In the midst of all this paranoia, I was not enjoying my children. In fact, I often had very little patience with them for no good reason. Little things they would do would just set me off and I would yell and scream at them to the point where I didn't even recognize myself. One morning, they were up really early shouting and playing very loudly. You know, just doing what kids do. Well, I must have been really tired that morning because I became furious, jumped out of bed, and quickly went into the other room where they were playing. With gritted teeth and a look of what I believe was pure lunacy, said, "Pleeeease beeeeee quieeeeeetttt!" My tone was hard to describe. It wasn't a yell, but more like a very forceful whisper, with a slight hint of crazy added to it. Startled for just a moment, the kids stopped what they were doing, looked at me oddly, and then started playing again. Go figure. I thought I must have been so scary to them. I know I was scary to myself. I'm just so grateful that I didn't traumatize my children. I'd like to think that they just thought Mommy was acting kooky - and I was, but to me, it was not in a good way. Sometimes Brad even had to tell me to step away from a situation and calm down whenever I was clearly over-reacting about something the kids did or were doing.

Granted, yes, lots of mothers lose their tempers and go through this with raising their children simply out of mere exhaustion, but for me, it was more than that. It almost felt like sometimes I was just going through the motions. I can't pinpoint exactly when it started, but somewhere along the way, I was not enjoying motherhood. I feel SO awful just saying that. It didn't make one bit of sense especially after everything we've been through with Maddy. I should have been embracing my wonderful children, but instead, it felt like I was pushing them away. It wasn't right. My kids mean everything to me and I wasn't appreciating them. I felt like a horrible, horrible mother. Perhaps the stresses and heartaches of the past years caught up with me and hardened me to a certain extent. Maybe this behavior was born out of the pressures I was under taking care of my son. I really don't know. All I know was that no amount of stress or frustration justified the way I sometimes behaved in front of my kids. This was not me and certainly not who I wanted to be. To be fair, I was not always like this, flying off the handle all willy nilly. In fact, it was really only a handful of times that I lost my temper and acted crazy, but for me, even if I did it only once, it would have been one time too many. Thankfully, at their young ages, I don't think the kids ever really noticed. My kids are the world to me and they deserved more and better than what I was giving them.

Chapter Fifty

With letting so many of fears take hold of me and with me taking my kids for granted, I felt like I was wasting this precious life. On more than one occasion I found myself sitting on the couch watching TV thinking, "What if something happens to me, won't I regret living life this way?" I kept having this internal dialogue with myself saying, "What if something happens to you? What if something happens to you?" I knew I was letting my fears and "issues" get in the way of being happy or living in the moment. I would beat myself up with these thoughts. Then all of a sudden, lo and behold, something did fucking happen! The other shoe fell. I got breast cancer. I couldn't believe it. Despite all of my efforts to follow superstitions and live life so carefully based on them, something bad happened anyway. How crazy is that?! I spent all of this energy being afraid of the unknown, afraid of things that didn't exist except in my own overactive imagination. Now there I was faced with a very, very real fear - cancer.

Perhaps in all of this, there was a higher power at work. Was this God's or the universe's way of telling me that I needed to make some serious changes in my life? It sure felt like it and I wasn't about to ignore it. I thought, "Could this be one of those blessings in disguise?" You're probably thinking, "How in the world could getting breast cancer possibly be a blessing?" For starters, it made me take a very hard look at myself. Ever since being diagnosed, I vowed to change for the better and appreciate every moment of every day, doing everything I could to not let my fears get the best of me. Granted, it is definitely a work in progress. Whenever I catch myself reverting back to old habits, I take note and make every effort to change my behavior for the best. I may not always succeed, but I sure as hell am trying.

The biggest change that I have made is with my kids. I have more patience, more kindness, and more love to give to them. I hug and kiss them so much more, and this time there is so much meaning behind each hug and each kiss. I hate that it took getting breast cancer to make me open my eyes and realize that I was missing out on so many wonderful moments with my children. As I said, a part of me believes it was a blessing in disguise. As horrible as it was to hear the "c" word, it made me reevaluate the way I was living my life and forced me to make some much needed changes, especially when it came to my children.

I have so much more patience with my kids when they misbehave and I handle things much more calmly at the little mischievous things that they do. I look back at those days when I was so quick to lose my temper with the kids and wonder how I could have ever let that happen. Some people would say to give myself a break, and that I was dealing with a lot, but I have a hard time forgiving myself for not being a better mom to my kids during that time. I have many regrets about the way I sometimes behaved, but I am enthusiastically making up for it. Maddox and Danika are my pride and joy. They are my heart. Motherhood is one of life's greatest gifts and I honor it every day by being the best mom that I know I can be to my children.

Often, I would watch the kids playing and just be in awe of them. They are so funny and often say the most insightful things. I find myself so much more aware of the many wondrous details of their emerging personalities. Sometimes I catch myself just staring at them and each time, I would fall more in love. I just want to take these moments all in. Soak it all up. Maddox and Danika are growing up to be such kind, caring, generous, compassionate, and loving human beings. I look at them and I know for a sure fact that I did something good in this world. Nothing is more important to me than being their Mommy.

As I geared up for my own battle, all I want is to survive, to be here for my kids for a very long time.

Chapter Fifty-One

I often think to myself, "Why did it have to take breast cancer for me to make these changes? Why did I have to get sick to face and work through my issues? Why couldn't I have been strong enough or courageous enough to overcome my fears on my own then maybe this wouldn't have happened?" These were some of the questions that I struggled with as I came to terms with my breast cancer diagnosis. As they say, hindsight is everything. One thing that I do know for sure is that I am a changed person because of it. I know that I am a better mother, a better wife, and a better person. As horrific as being diagnosed with breast cancer was, it has undeniably given me a whole new outlook on life and how to live it. The way you live life is with everything you have. I learned the hard way that as much as I tried, I couldn't control everything. All I can do is embrace all that is good in every moment, and take absolutely nothing for granted. I prayed this attitude would hold strong and serve me well in the coming months. As I prepared to embark on the challenging journey ahead of me, I knew that my courage and strength would be tested. What I didn't realize yet, was just how much.

Chapter Fifty-Two

This is what I understood from the biopsy. The breast cancer was diagnosed as Invasive Ductal Carcinoma. The tumor was localized and fairly small. Based on the mammogram, it was around 1.4 cm so it was considered Stage 1. I caught it early. Thank God. This information was reassuring. I would know more once I met with the surgeons to discuss a plan of action. The thing with scheduling an appointment just to get consultations with some of these breast surgeons, particularly in Manhattan, is that it takes a long time to book it, some as far as one to two months away. All I wanted was to get this thing out of me, like yesterday! I would soon learn that there would be a lot of waiting with this process - waiting to get the biopsy report, waiting for the consultation, waiting to get the surgery, waiting to get the pathology. You really get a lot of practice in patience.

I scheduled consultations with two surgeons so that I could get two opinions, one from Mount Sinai and the other from Sloan Kettering. I really didn't feel the need to consider other facilities. I had enough experience with my son having gone to both places that those were my top picks. One appointment took two weeks to get and the other took 4 weeks. Waiting for these appointments was excruciating. It felt like the longest time because I was very aware of walking around with this "thing" inside me.

When I finally met with the first surgeon, she explained that I was a good candidate for a lumpectomy because the tumor was small and localized. Since I have no family history of breast cancer, she believed a mastectomy was not necessary. She went on to explain that a lumpectomy would be followed by radiation, and depending on the pathology of the tumor, chemo may also be recommended. When she mentioned chemo, I disregarded it. I remember thinking - Stage 1, small tumor, I'm not going to need chemo. I didn't even factor it in. For some reason, it didn't really even scare me. All I can say now is that I was incredibly naive.

The second surgeon also gave me the same recommendation for the lumpectomy. Both surgeons explained the importance of clean margins, which meant getting all the cancer out, and also checking the lymph nodes during surgery, to make sure the cancer did not spread. Once I had all the information, I made the decision to get a lumpectomy at Sloan Kettering. Sloan was also where my son was getting his treatment so it was an easy decision, and one that made the most sense. I also had a good feeling about this surgeon. She was kind and had a very warm and easy way about her, and more importantly, I trusted her to do the procedure. It all seemed pretty simple as I really didn't think beyond the surgery. My main thoughts were focused on getting clean margins and clean lymph nodes. The surgery was scheduled and I figured once the tumor was out, that would be that. I was a little scared, but I was mostly relieved that it would soon be out of me.

In the weeks before the surgery, it was a strange feeling knowing I was walking around with this tumor in my breast. I tried to ignore it, but at the same time, I was very conscious of it. Sometimes I had the urge to just feel it and other times, like when I was in the shower, my hands wouldn't dare go near it. The surgery couldn't come soon enough.

Chapter Fifty-Three

While I waited to get the surgery, my doctor scheduled me for genetic testing. This is also the test that checks for BRCA, the breast cancer gene. I am not going to go too much into this topic because truth be told, I pretty much blocked it all out. It is basically a blood test, but before you get your blood drawn, they throw so much scary - and I mean *really* scary, information at you for like two hours. There was so much of - "this could happen or that could happen" - and none of it good! As I sat there listening to these various horrific scenarios, I made myself tune out much of it because it was freaking me out! I remember I just kept thinking, "I don't want to die. I don't want to die." They really made you fear for your life. They did not just put this fear in you, they were practically beating you over the head with it.

I think it was quite inconsiderate for them to go through so much detail on things that may not apply to you. For cancer patients who already have enough on their minds, why would you subject them to this plethora of frightening information until the lab results are in?! I get that they want the patients to be informed, but this was ridiculous. In my very strong opinion, they should draw your blood first, get the results, and then explain ONLY the things that pertain to you.

By the time they drew my blood, I was a hot frightened mess. While I never let them see me sweat, so to speak, I was mentally exhausted and so ready to be out of there. I can honestly tell you that I was truly traumatized by that appointment. I went home nearly in tears and very shaken up. I think it is incredibly insensitive and perhaps, even irresponsible, to put anyone through that until the labs are completed and all the facts are known.

Once all the reports were in, my results showed that I tested negative for both BRCA1 and BRCA2, with all the other tests normal. I wanted to get on my knees and pray, "Thank you sweet, Jesus." As you can imagine, I was beyond RELIEVED.

Chapter Fifty-Four

Surgery Day

This was a very straightforward outpatient procedure. My appointment was for 5:30AM which was great because then I knew my surgery would be one of the first ones scheduled. My husband and I arrived around 5:15AM. We both seemed pretty relaxed and ready. I wasn't really nervous about the surgery. I just wanted to get it done. After being prepped, my husband and I exchanged kisses and told each other that we loved each other. I was in the OR by 7:30AM. I said hello to the doctor, hopped on the operating table, and then all of a sudden, I felt very woozy. I didn't even notice any of the nurses fiddling with my IV. Nobody told me that they administered the anesthesia already. It worked so quickly. One minute I was talking to the doctor and the next minute, I was out!

I woke up from the surgery very groggy with very little pain and just some minor discomfort from the incision sites. I spoke with the surgeon briefly who told me that the surgery went well and that I was scheduled to meet with her in a week for the follow-up. I was glad to see my husband, and as soon as the grogginess wore off, we went home.

Recuperating from the lumpectomy was fairly easy. I wasn't in any real pain and never even needed the prescribed pain-killers. I had to wear a tight-fitting bra to keep the bandages in place. Since the lumpectomy was done on my left breast, it was a bit difficult to lift up my left arm for a while so taking a shower and getting dressed was sometimes tricky, but other than that, and some soreness, I was recovering well. I made sure my kids and my husband were very gentle with me.

At my follow-up the next week, my surgeon walked in the room and with a big smile said, "All good reports!" She told me that my lymph nodes are negative and that the margins are clear. I felt an overwhelming sense of relief. I thanked the Lord once again. She said the next step was for me to meet with the oncologist who would go over the pathology reports and discuss the treatment plan. I wasn't worried at that point and thought the meeting with the oncologist was just a formality. I was prepared to do the radiation treatment which is generally the protocol after a lumpectomy. From what I heard, radiation was a very simple procedure and that basically, all you do, to put it simply, is lie back and get zapped for a few seconds. The main inconvenience is that you have to do it every day for several weeks. I gave my surgeon a heartfelt hug and left feeling very confident that I could handle that.

Chapter Fifty-Five

It was about month after my lumpectomy that I had my meeting with the oncologist. Like my surgeon, she too seemed genuinely warm, caring, and friendly. I liked her right away. When I chose to go to Sloan Kettering, I didn't really have any referrals for doctors there, so I picked both my surgeon and my oncologist based on quite favorable patient reviews on the internet. Thankfully, after meeting them, the good reviews were pretty accurate.

My husband and kids came with me to the appointment. I'm not sure why we took the kids to this appointment, but there we all were. As the oncologist went through the pathology reports, I was not prepared for what she was about to tell me. She said the tumor that was removed was bigger than they initially thought and that the reports indicated that it was an aggressive tumor. Because of that information, she was recommending chemo. Oh, fuck. She said that the chemo would be a precautionary measure. I went to this appointment thinking that I would just be getting information about my radiation treatment. Now, I had to get chemo too? I calmed myself inside and took a moment in my mind to absorb all of this. For some unknown reason, I thought, "Well, how hard could it be?" Boy, was I a dummy. I remember just sitting there and not really reacting. I can't remember whether I was in shock or whether I was just under the delusion that it'll be okay, that I can get through the chemo with little discomfort. I think I even, for the very briefest of moments, thought about how cool it would be to wear some wigs. How ridiculous is that?! I was so foolish.

The doctor explained that there were three options of chemo treatments: mild, moderate, and strong. Because I was young and physically fit, she was recommending the strongest treatment. Oh fuck, fuck. I had no clue what this meant at the time, but it sounded serious. I was processing so much information that I made myself try to hold back any emotional response. I sat there with my husband and my children listening to the doctor talk about recurrence and mortality rates. I couldn't believe I was talking about *mortality* rates. Once again, I thought, "Oh my God, I don't want to die!" There I was talking to the doctor in front of my family, in front of my children, about survival rates! For the first time since hearing about chemo, I was really scared. I felt my pulse begin to quicken and did my best to keep it together. She talked about some of the risks with chemo, some of which were quite frightening to say the least. She continued on explaining some of the possible side effects like nausea and hair loss. I tried to tune the scary parts out which was not an easy task. With each bit of information, I felt this fear building inside me and wanting to take over, but I willed myself to suppress it. As you may have already surmised, I often tend to operate on the idea that ignorance is bliss, so I do have a tendency to block out things that I don't want to hear. It's my defense mechanism. Self Preservation. Once again, I would rely on my husband to get the details while I took in only the information that I could handle emotionally.

The doctor had her recommendation to do the strongest treatment, but ultimately it would be my choice. I didn't want to do the strongest one, but I was also afraid that the mild one would not be as effective. Who was I, freakin' Goldilocks?! Somehow I knew picking the one that was "just right" was not going to be as easy for me as it was for Goldi. I also had to factor in the possible risks associated with each chemo treatment. Geez. Step right up, pick your poison. There was always the option of not doing any chemo at all, but the doctor strongly advised against that. I felt like I was gambling with my life. I heard someone once say that having a choice doesn't always mean having control. I think for anyone faced with this decision, the thought of having little to no control over what happens is probably the hardest and scariest things to accept. It was all so surreal. There I was sitting next to my husband processing all of this as my kids innocently watched a cartoon video, blissfully unaware of why we were there. Meanwhile, I was faced to make the decision of my life - literally.

There was one more test that I took called the onco-type test, which basically is an indicator of whether chemo would be of any benefit. The results could also show whether chemo would not be recommended. It was kind of that last piece of the puzzle that I needed on whether or not it would be to my advantage to get chemo. At the time of this appointment, my results were not in yet for this test so the doctor suggested that we wait for the results to come in before I make a decision on my treatment plan. We went home and I immediately took to the internet to research each of the chemo "cocktails" in the hopes that it would help me make a decision. As much as I was desperate for information, I was also very careful to gloss over any parts that scared me. I was thankful for my husband who read every detail. He was my shield giving me a filtered version of all the research. There are some people that want to know every single detail. I am not that person. The less I know, the better. I have a very overactive imagination and I tend to overthink things so I know that it was in my best interest to just stick with the basics. Of course, I wanted to make an informed and thoughtful decision, but not at the expense of my sanity. Once I read what I felt was sufficient information, I moved on. I also consulted with some friends, some of whom are breast cancer survivors themselves. Their opinions varied, with some opting for the strongest treatment, while others recommended the holistic route with no chemo at all.

My husband was very strong throughout this whole process. I'm not really sure what was going on in his head or with his emotions as we dealt with cancer for the second time. If he was scared, which I'm sure he was, he never let me know it. We did our best to approach all the information and all the statistics from the doctor, and from our research, like it was all business.

My mother-in-law called me that afternoon to find out how my appointment went with the oncologist. I told her how the doctor was recommending chemo and not just any chemo, but the strongest one. All of a sudden, as I heard myself actually say it, I finally broke down. It surprised me. Of course throughout this process, I've gotten emotional and have certainly teared up, but this was the first time I had a full out cry since I was diagnosed with breast cancer. Somehow hearing me talk about chemo out loud made it even more real. I realized in that moment, that choosing a chemo treatment was certainly not "all business," it was very, very personal.

I went to bed that night still unsure of which treatment plan to choose. I didn't know what to do. I lay there with all of this information and all of these emotions just swirling around inside me. I felt a sadness come over me that night. Was this really happening? All I wanted was to grow old with my husband and to be here to watch Maddox and Danika have families of their own. For any mother battling cancer, one of the greatest fears is not being there for your children. My heart ached with this fear. No one would love my kids as much as I do. No one would take care of my kids the way I do. I wanted to hold them and never let go. Everything seemed so fragile. As these thoughts consumed me, all I could do was pray as I wept silently in the night. Please God, let me be a mother to my children.

The next day, I got the onco-type results. Drum roll, please. The score was 21. Wouldn't you know it, the score fell in the grey zone. Yep, the freakin' grey zone. I guess I thought this score was going to help me make a decision. Instead, it left me with more questions. Scoring in the grey zone basically meant that there was no way to tell whether chemo would benefit me. As if the decision wasn't hard enough before, now do I consider the mild option or perhaps do I consider to not do chemo at all? Previously, my doctor felt very strongly about recommending the stronger treatment, but in light of this score, she said that I could go with any of the three treatment plans. That being said, she also advised against not doing any chemo at all. A part of me was relieved that I scored in the grey zone because it gave me what I thought was a valid reason for not going with the strongest treatment. After all, there is something to be said about not wanting to be over-treated. So I guess in a way, the score did help narrow down my choices. After lots of very careful consideration, and based on all the information we had, my husband and I decided on the moderate chemo plan. We discussed this in detail with my doctor and with her blessing and support, we felt confident in our decision.

Chapter Fifty-Six

January 19, 2012

Go Time. This was the day of my first cycle of chemo. I was to get my treatment at the Evelyn H. Lauder Breast Center. In the moderate chemo plan there would be four cycles of chemo, with each cycle three weeks apart. It was a cocktail of two drugs, Taxotere and cyclophosphamide, also known as Cytoxan. It would be administered through an IV. These cycles would be followed by a shot called Neulasta, given the next day in order to boost my white blood count. That was the drill.

I prepared myself as best as I could for this day. As I waited in the sitting room to be called in, I gazed at all the women in the room. Some women wore scarves or caps, some wore their wigs, and others were just plain bald - and brave. I took it in and felt sad for all of them, for all of us, that we had to go through this. I noticed that most of the women appeared much older and it struck me how I was one of the youngest women there. I felt out of place and questioned how this could have happened to me. Let's face it, cancer sucks at any age, but at 40 years old, I was blindsided by this. As I looked around the room, I noticed there was one other younger woman there with her family. She may actually have been younger than me. She had her daughter with her who maybe was barely one year old. This woman had a cap on so I knew her hair had already fallen off. I watched her with her daughter on her lap and thought about how strong this woman must be to be taking care of such a young child while going through chemo. I admired her. I forced back tears as I thought about my own kids and how much I loved them. I wanted to be brave for my children, like this woman was for her daughter. Sitting there, I couldn't help but be moved by all of these courageous women. Their fight was now my fight too.

As my name was called to go in, all I thought was - let's just get this over with so that I can get to the next cycle, and the next, until I'm done! The facilities were very simple and nice, and my room was private with its own TV and lots of natural light, with windows looking out into the city streets. I watched all of the people outside going about their business seemingly without a care in the world, while I was in this room preparing myself for chemo. It didn't seem real. I envied the people outside and gave myself permission, for just a moment, to feel sorry for myself. This really sucks.

My husband was there for moral support. He sat with me while the nurse explained the chemo process. I was nervous. As the nurse got everything ready, the mood in the room was very subdued. It was time to get started. I winced a little as she inserted the IV needle in arm. With my husband by my side, I sat there quietly, closed my eyes, and took a deep breath as I got my first infusion of chemo. As these drugs entered my body, I willed them to kill any cancer, just like I willed it to do the same when Maddy started his chemo. I willed my body to protect itself against this poison while it did its job. At some point, I remember slightly shivering feeling very cold and was given a blanket. Every so often, the nurse came in to check on how I was doing. Aside from getting chemo, I was peachy. After a while, I felt okay to be there by myself. There was no reason for my husband to stay for the whole process, so he left early to pick the kids up from school. I did my best to just focus on anything but what was happening. I watched TV as a distraction and after maybe two or three hours, the infusions were done. Cycle One - check.

The nurse informed me of some possible side effects and gave me a list of over-the- counter vitamins that I should take. She also gave me several prescriptions for nausea. In fact, she gave me three prescriptions for nausea - each one had varied strengths depending on how sick I got. Great.

I chose to start the cycles on Thursdays, rather than the other option which was to start on Mondays. Starting on Thursdays would allow me to have the whole weekend to rest and recover as needed. I went home that first Thursday very aware of my body. I felt like I was in a constant state of anticipation. I wondered when I would experience the side effects, if any, of these drugs. In the meantime, I went about my day as usual, taking care of the kids, doing household chores, and making dinner. I went to bed that night and thought, "Okay, day one, not bad."

Friday, the next morning, was a school day. My husband took the day off to look after me as we really didn't know what to expect. We dropped the kids off at school and went out for breakfast. It was then that I felt the first side effect. Sitting there at the table, I noticed that my fingers started to tingle. It was subtle at first, but then it became more obvious. It wasn't painful and didn't cause any major discomfort, but there it was. I knew this was one of the side effects of one of the drugs. They already prepared me for this by instructing me to take B vitamins which I believe was supposed to ease that side effect. That afternoon, I got my Neulasta shot. I braced myself for the rest of the day, wondering what side effect I would experience next, but as the afternoon and evening came of that day, nothing. Again, I said to myself, "Wow. This isn't too bad. I can handle this."

Chapter Fifty-Seven

Up until this point, only my family and a handful of people knew what was going on with me. I was extremely private about this. We've been through so much already with Maddox and then to have this happen to me, I wasn't ready to share my news with anybody. I knew what they'd be thinking and feeling. I didn't want to say anything because I hated the thought of anyone feeling sorry for me or our family. It was unimaginable that both my son and I were getting chemo at the same time. Somehow my husband convinced me that it was time to share my news so that if we needed help while I was on chemo, I'd have friends that I can call upon for support. So that day, I sent an e-mail out to my closest girlfriends and gave them the news. It felt like deja vu. It wasn't that long ago that I was sending a similar message to our friends telling them about Maddox. Now it was about me.

On January 20, 2012, I sent this e-mail. This is what I wrote:

Hi Ladies,

As some of my closest friends, I wanted to share this information with you. In October of 2011, I was diagnosed with breast cancer. I had a successful lumpectomy in November and I am now in a treatment plan of chemo, radiation, and hormone therapy. I am doing well and looking at this situation as an opportunity to make changes in my life for the better.

I know your first instinct is to call me and I love you all for that. It can be overwhelming and emotional to talk about it at times, so I will respond to your e-mails and we will talk another time.

In the beginning, I wanted to handle this privately as I hated the thought of anyone feeling sorry for me. I realize now that I had to get over it and look at the bigger picture. If I can be play a small part in creating more awareness for this disease among women, I believe it is my obligation to share this information with all of you.

I found my lump doing a very random self-breast exam in the shower. I was truly in disbelief when I felt it. I was in even more disbelief when they told me I had early stages of breast cancer. Even now, it is kind of unimaginable that both my son and I are cancer patients. With that said, it is my brave five year old son that has taught me a thing or two about courage and resilience. Because of that we are both strong on our journeys towards good health.

I am writing all of you to share my story, but especially to urge all of you to get screening mammograms or do monthly self- breast exams. At the very least, know what "normal" feels like for your breast so you know when something feels different. I do not say any of this to scare you, but for you to know you can take charge of your good health. Breast Cancer Awareness is there to empower women. When I found out, I was very scared, but ultimately I was even more thankful that it was caught early and I am now taking important steps to conquer it.

So I will not let C stand for cancer. For me, it will stand for CURE. It will stand for COURAGE and it will stand for how CUTE I will look in my wigs :) I may throw in a couple of sexy styles for Brad. He is amazing through all of this so I figured he should get some perks!

Power to my beautiful sistas!

Love you guys,
~ Geri

Needless to say, just like with Maddy, the outpouring of support was immediate. I received so many e-mails and messages of love and encouragement. I was overcome with emotion with each and every note. Some offered to sit with me through the chemo, others offered to baby-sit so that I could rest, many offered to provide food, and the others simply told me how much they loved me. I cried with each and every thoughtful message. It was too much, but at the same time, it was what I needed. Even now as I remember some of those messages, I am brought to tears. In my own time, I responded to each them, mostly through e-mail because I felt so very fragile. I knew I wouldn't be able to keep it together on the phone hearing their voices and mine. I knew I could write to them, but I wasn't quite ready to talk about it. For now, it was enough that they knew. I went to bed that night strengthened by the love and support of my family and friends. I would soon need it.

Chapter Fifty-Eight

Saturday came and the tingling in my fingers was barely
noticeable. What I did notice by that evening was just a hint of a
strange metallic taste in my mouth. I was able to eat my dinner,
but it definitely tasted very different. That night, I also felt a slight
urinary irritation, similar to a UTI, urinary tract infection. I was
aware that that was one of the possible side effects of the Cytozan
drug. This side effect seemed minor and I went to bed again
actually thinking, "This is manageable."

Then along came Sunday. This fourth day hit me like a ton of
bricks. I woke up in extreme discomfort from the urinary
irritation. If you've ever had a urinary tract infection, you know it
can be terribly painful. This sensation felt like a UTI. There was
that urgency to go to the bathroom frequently and when you do go,
it is just a trickle, with this horrendous burning sensation. It is
awful. I thought drinking a lot of water would flush it out, but it
didn't work. As the day progressed, so did the discomfort, so
much so that I had to phone the on-call nurse. She instructed me to
go to the ER so they could run some tests. Well, of course it was
freezing and snowing outside. I knew I'd be there for hours
getting these tests and then probably spend more hours waiting for
the results. The last thing I wanted to do was go out and get
examined, but the pain was getting close to unbearable. So I
trudged out in the wintry mess. To add insult to injury, that
metallic taste I had the night before only got worse and I barely
had anything to eat because everything literally tasted like paper.
With that said, I did not have any nausea. I guess be thankful for
small favors.

There I was, at the ER, getting my blood drawn and examined. My
veins tend to hide so it is not the easiest thing to get my blood
drawn. Lots of times, they have to draw it from my hand. This
particular nurse was not gentle with the needle. She tried my arm,
but couldn't get the vein, so then she went for the hand. I
remember getting poked all over the place and her moving the
needle around while it was in my hand to get to the vein! It really

hurt. I had a horrible flashback to when Maddy was poked mercilessly with needles before he got his port. It's awful to think that my son had to endure such pain. To say that it was an unpleasant experience for either of us would be an understatement.

As I figured, I waited several hours before the results came in. When they finally did, the report showed that it was not a UTI. I couldn't believe it. It felt exactly like a UTI, but the doctor explained that it was most likely the Cytozan that was causing the bladder irritation. There was nothing left to do but go home and ride it out. I went home praying for some relief. Thankfully, as evening came, the urinary pain eased up and by the Monday morning, the bladder irritation was gone. I barely had a moment's peace before the nausea hit me that same morning. It suddenly felt like my body was being assaulted from all of these directions. I would get over one side effect only to be slammed by another one.

Similar to the other side effects, the nausea was very mild at first. Although I felt queasy, I was able to bring my kids to school without any incident - thank goodness. It was a huge relief to have the kids in school so that I can just sit and ride out this nausea by myself at home. Good thing too because the nausea was increasing by the moment. I remember literally just sitting on the couch for what may have been several hours, with my eyes closed, taking deep breaths to curb the queasiness. I was hungry, but still could barely eat anything because of that metallic taste in my mouth. Between that nasty taste and the nausea, my appetite was shot. I forced myself to munch on crackers to just have something in my stomach. I knew I had that anti-nausea medication in the cupboard, but call me crazy, I really wanted to avoid taking it. I just felt that there were enough drugs in my system that I didn't want to add any more to it than I had too. Well by that afternoon, I had too. I could only hold off wanting to vomit for so long. I decided to take the mildest of the medications. I'm not sure that it made any difference because although the urge to vomit subsided hours later, I still felt an underlying queasiness all day. At least I managed to pick up my kids from school, but made them walk quickly home just in case their mommy had to bow down to the porcelain throne. I moved very slowly the rest of the day and despite that icky taste in my mouth, I forced myself to eat some kind of dinner.

That night I noticed a slight rash on my back and hands. My hands sometimes get these mild rashes during the winter due to severe dryness so I thought nothing of it at first. The only thing that was unusual was that there was a rash on a small section of my back. One of chemo pamphlets did mention to notify the doctor if any rashes developed. I showed the rashes to my husband and he agreed that I should call the nurse in the morning. Without any further thought of it, I was more than ready to call it a day.

Chapter Fifty-Nine

I woke up Tuesday morning feeling okay. The nausea seemed to have subsided a bit. I called the nurse to let her know about the rashes thinking it would be nothing. She told me that it could be an allergic reaction to the Taxotere. Oh, nooooo! When she said that, I began to worry. I asked her what would happen if I was allergic. She said that the doctor would have options for that. What kind of options??? One of my major concerns was that the first cycle would have to be done again or worse, that I'd have to change treatment plans. The nurse reassured me that whatever the doctor decided, it would not in any way extend my treatment an extra cycle. While that was somewhat comforting, one thing I knew for sure was that I did not want to change the treatment plan. I had already started it and I really didn't want to make any changes to the drugs I was already administered. The nurse instructed me to take a picture of the rashes on my hand and e-mail them to her so that she can show them to my doctor. She said she'd follow up with me that day.

Since I was actually feeling up to it, I went to the gym. Before I began my treatment, I promised myself that I would continue to exercise on the days that I felt good. I was there for about thirty minutes when the nurse called me back. She told me that my doctor wanted me to have the rashes looked at by a specialist as soon as possible in case it was an allergic reaction to one of the chemo drugs. The nurse had already made the appointment and asked me to leave right away. It was something that had to be looked at in person. My heart sank. I had already spent most of Sunday at the ER and now this. Reluctantly, I left the gym and got ready for yet another examination.

My mother-in-law was arriving that afternoon to stay with us for a few days to help while I was on chemo. Thankfully, she would be able to pick up the kids from school in case I was held up at the doctor's office getting this freakin' rash looked at. I remember sitting in another exam room, staring at the floor, feeling depressed. Why oh why couldn't I just get through the first cycle of chemo without any issues? Ha! Foolish, foolish girl. The doctor examined the rashes and told me that they would have to do a biopsy to determine whether it is indeed an allergic reaction to the chemo. It would involve cutting a sample of the skin on my back at the rash site. Son of a bitch. You gotta be fucking kidding me. They prepped me for the incision and bent my upper body forward to get easy access to the site. As I dropped my head forward and felt the cut, I started crying. I felt powerless. Thank goodness I was bent down so no one could tell that I was in tears. The incision hurt, but I wasn't crying from the physical pain. I was crying because I felt like a specimen getting poked, and cut, and examined, over and over again. I had had enough and it was only my first cycle.

After the examination, the doctor was able to get my oncologist on the phone with her to discuss the findings. With me in the room, I heard her tell my oncologist that the reaction seemed mild because it was only on my hands and back, and that because it didn't appear until 4 to 5 days after the infusion, that they could "rechallenge" the drugs. "Rechallenge?!" Say what now? I was like, "Hello, excuse me, I am sitting right here! Don't I have a say?!" It sounded like they were "challenging" these drugs to a duel or something, with me as the unwilling opponent. No thank you! As you can imagine, I did not appreciate that choice of word, "rechallenge." They say what doesn't kill you makes you stronger. Hmp, for the moment, I had a hard time believing that. I didn't know what was going to happen. All I knew was that I just wanted to get the hell of there. I wanted to go home! The doctor said they should have the results of the biopsy the next day and she would discuss the next course of action with my oncologist. Terrific.

That night as I was preparing dinner for my kids, my mind was in a different place. I felt physically and mentally exhausted, but more than that, I felt a deep sense of despair. My mother-in-law came into the kitchen and I broke down. I couldn't stop the tears. She held my hand as I told her how I was so tired of going from one doctor to another, and how I hated all of this poking and being examined. I felt so defeated. I thought of Maddox and it brought back memories of those early days when he was diagnosed. I remembered all too well how he too was subjected to needles, x-rays, and tests. I had images of watching my son crying in fear and pain getting needles placed in his arm as my husband and I were helpless to stop it. I thought if I, a grown woman, was going through all of this anguish, I can't even imagine how traumatic it must have been for a two year old boy. He was just a baby. It breaks my heart all over again to remember that he had to go through all of that. I was in awe of him. There I was complaining about all of this and there was my son, my brave, brave boy who put everything into perspective. Get it together, girl. And I did. My son gave me courage because he had courage. It was me and Maddy against the world. We each had our own battle to fight and we were going to fight it with everything we had.

The next day my oncologist called me and said that the biopsy did show signs of an allergic reaction to the drugs, most likely the Taxotere. She agreed with the specialist that since it was a somewhat mild response, and because it didn't show up until several days after the infusion, she felt that we could "rechallenge" the drugs and continue with the treatment plan. There was that word again. As much as it was my preference to stick with the same treatment plan, I asked her whether it would be dangerous to continue on the same drugs since I did indeed have an allergic reaction to one of them. There I was, waiting for her to say, "Of course not, we would not do it if it were dangerous." Instead, she paused, and this is what she says, "Well, there are always risks with chemo." Are you serious?! What the hell does that mean?! In that moment, I remembered a conversation I had with friend, who also had breast cancer. She told me that chemo could kill you. Nice friend, huh. Actually, she is a close friend, and while I appreciated her tell-it-like-it-is attitude, I could have really used some sugar coating. Same goes for my doctor. I know, I know. It's better to know the truth. Well, fuck that. What I really wanted was for my doctor to tell me that there was nothing to worry about. I guess she must have realized that I was on the verge of freaking out because she went on to explain how she would take several precautions with the second cycle. She would make sure that I was monitored very closely every step of the way during the infusions.

I was relieved that we weren't making any changes to my treatment, but at the same time, I was already bracing myself for the second round. Ultimately, I of course respected my doctor for telling me the truth, but that doesn't mean that she still didn't scare the hell out of me. All I could do was trust my doctor. God help me.

Chapter Sixty

By mid week, my body felt like it was easing from the drugs. The only side effect that lingered was the slight queasiness and metallic taste in my mouth, which consequently made it very difficult to have a proper meal. By the weekend, the nausea was gone and food tasted normal again. I was so thankful to enjoy food the way it was meant to taste!

When I started treatment, the nurse explained to me that the roughest days would start around the second day after the infusion, and that I should start feeling the upswing by the fifth day. She explained that any nausea I experienced in the first cycle should be consistent with the rest of the cycles. I really hated the nausea, but I guess it was good to know that after a week, based on this first cycle, that the nausea does dissipate. Knowing this made it seem more manageable.

One of the major side effects of chemo is fatigue. Unlike the nausea, the nurse said that this side effect would be cumulative, which meant that with each cycle, I would get more and more tired. She went on to say that this fatigue would be very different from your typical tiredness. She said that usually when you are tired, you get some rest, and then you feel re-energized. With the extreme fatigue caused by chemo, you can rest all day, but your body will feel like it never rested at all, that it would still feel the exhaustion. During this first cycle, I don't recall feeling very tired. Perhaps it was because I was so distracted dealing with the other side effects that I didn't notice being more tired than usual.

By the middle of the second week after my first infusion, I felt like myself again. I would have about a week of that good feeling before getting hit with the second round.

Chapter Sixty-One

The Hair

I knew the hair loss would be happening soon. I was told that the hair starts falling out right around two weeks after the first cycle. They were correct. I have to say that I was not very emotional or upset about my hair falling out. It was very different with my son. Many people told us that we may want to consider getting my son's hair shaved before it actually started falling out because it can be very traumatic watching it happen. As I mentioned, the interesting thing with Maddox was that it took a very long time for his hair to fall out. Whenever we would go to one of his check-ups, the nurses and doctors were amazed that he still had his hair. Of course eventually it did fall out, but his hair hung on for a pretty long time.

I wasn't sure whether it would be the same for me - whether my hair would hang strong. Nevertheless, I certainly was not running to get my head shaved. As I approached that momentous week, I did find it kind of odd that I wasn't getting very emotional about the hair. I remembered a conversation that my mother-in-law and I had when Maddy's hair fell out. She wondered whether Maddy got upset about losing his hair. We both agreed that he was unaware about the whole thing. As a three year boy at the time, he was too young to comprehend what was happening, let alone care about having no hair. My mother-in-law then said it would be very different for an adult, especially a woman, to have to experience that. Two years later, *I* was that woman. Unbelievable, huh. Yet, there I was, preparing for that very thing. A part of me felt ready for it to fall out, and it's possible that an even bigger part of me may have detached myself from the situation.

Well, ready or not, the day came. I was in the bathroom totally not thinking that this was the day, much less *the* moment that it would happen. I casually ran my fingers through my hair and there it was, right in front of me, a handful of strands at the palm of my hand. I didn't cry. I don't even think I freaked out. All I remember was that I gagged just a tiny bit. For real. I know it was a strange reaction, but that's what happened. I didn't dare brush my hair for the rest of the day.

As the week passed, there was no stopping it. I would take a shower and just lightly shampoo my hair in an effort to keep it place, but every time, I would look in the drain and there would be tons of hair. I would get up from the couch and notice strands and strands of hair on the cushions. I would put the very little hair I had left in a ponytail and every day, I noticed it getting thinner and thinner. I knew I was prolonging the inevitable, but I just wasn't ready to part with my hair just yet. I guess I was more "attached" to it than I realized. Eventually though, I let my husband cut it as short as it could be, without completely shaving it all off. I donated what little hair he managed to cut to an organization that makes wigs for cancer patients. For a couple of days, I just had a really, really short haircut. However, even those tiny hairs couldn't hang on, and so one night, I finally allowed my husband to shave my head.

As I saw what was left of my hair fall to the ground, I felt at peace with it. When the deed was done, it actually looked okay, dare I say, even good - not Demi Moore, G.I. Jane good, but good enough for me. The true test was showing my kids. Initially, I had explained to them that Mommy was taking medicine that was going to make her hair fall out. They didn't quite understand, but they knew that Mommy's hair was going to be very short. That evening I prepared to show Maddox and Danika my new "look." They were sitting in the dining room and I came in with a cap on my head and said, "Are you ready to see Mommy's new hair-do?" I guess I should have said "no-hair" do. They both shouted together, "YEAH!" I took a deep breath and watched their excited faces light up as I slowly took my cap off. Danika, as honest as kids are at that age, says, "Mommy, I like your hair better longer." I laughed and replied, "Me too, girl." Then I looked at my son and he says, "You look beautiful, Mommy." I teared up at the sincerity and sweetness of my little boy and that was all I needed to hear to hold my bald head up high.

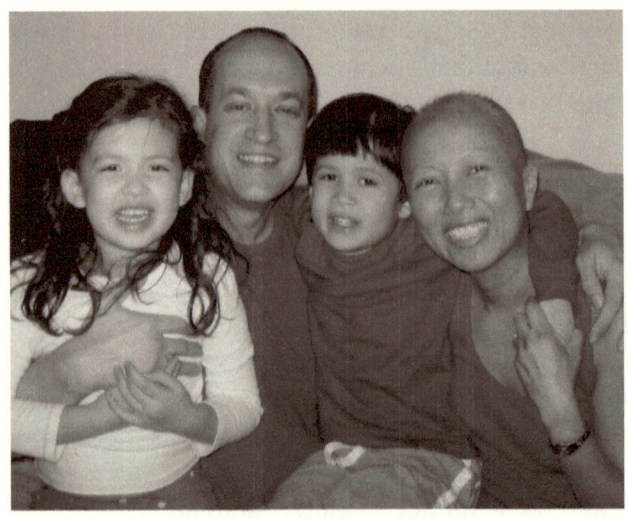

"You look beautiful, Mommy."

While, I kept my look au natural at home, I did have several wigs on the ready and no one was the wiser. One of the wigs was a baseball cap that had hair strategically placed on it. That was the best. It was easy on, easy off. That became my go to piece whenever I had to run a quick errand or pick my kids up from school. I also had a wig that looked very natural and casual. It was a shoulder length bob with bangs. Before the hair fell out, everyone knew me with long hair. I had a couple of the moms at school compliment me on my new "haircut" when they saw me with this wig on for the first time. Oh, if they only knew.

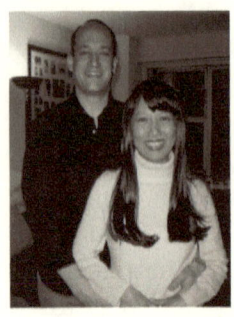
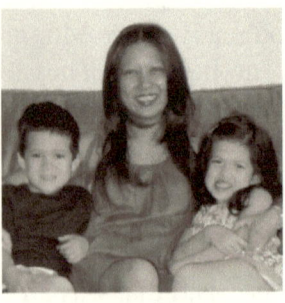
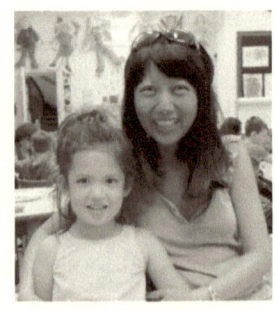

Date Night Wig.   Fancy Wig.   Casual Wig.

There was actually only one mom that knew that I had breast cancer and was undergoing chemo. I just didn't feel the need to share it with anyone else from the school, and I certainly did not want it to become public knowledge. Because of that, I often found myself rushing to leave after picking up my kids so that I could avoid any conversation. Usually at pick-up, all of the parents and nannies form a line outside the classroom waiting for the kids' dismissal. It was during that wait on line that we would engage in conversation. The moms would bond and plan play dates. Those minutes before dismissal were tough for me because I was either feeling crummy from the chemo and just didn't want to chat, or I was afraid someone would mention the hair and I would have to lie and casually say that I just cut it. Every time I was afraid that they would realize it was a wig. It made me feel so uncomfortable to blatantly lie to people and chat with them as if nothing was going on with me. So I just put a smile on my face, politely said my hellos, and basically kept to myself, doing my best to avoid any socialization.

When I look back at those times, I feel a little regret that I wasn't able to join in the friendships that the other moms were obviously making. I just felt very self-conscious. I was friendly, but I definitely had a wall up. Brad also took the kids to most of the birthday parties. Many of those times, I was just not in any shape to take them myself. I get sad that I missed out on all of those fun occasions with my kids. Those were also more opportunities to bond with other parents, but I was just not up to it both physically and emotionally. It's very possible that many of the parents thought I was being anti-social, when really, I was just trying to be private about having chemo treatment. I don't blame them if they did think that because for the most part, I was anti-social, but it wasn't because I wanted to be, it was because my circumstances made me that way.

Chapter Sixty-Two

Ding! Round Two

As you can imagine, I was particularly apprehensive about this second cycle. I wasn't sure what to expect and that was the scariest thing. Because I had experienced some kind of allergic reaction, they planned to do a much slower infusion. The doctor also added an extra bag of saline to the infusions in order to alleviate the bladder irritation I had gotten with the first cycle. This was going to be a long day.

For some reason, both my husband and my kids were there with me for this second cycle. I'm thinking it must have been because Brad wanted to be there with me, and since we didn't have a babysitter that day, we just decided to take the kids with us. The kids must not have had school, or perhaps my appointment was later in the afternoon. I can't quite remember. I'm guessing that it had to have been one of those reasons because having my kids watch me get chemo was not something I would have allowed or otherwise, wanted. In any event, we were all in my treatment room while the nurse explained all the precautions they were going to take with this cycle. As my kids watched me get my IV put in, I remember telling my son, Maddox, that I was going to be brave, just like him when he gets his "medicine." The next thing I know, the nurse is telling me that it may be best for the kids to be in the waiting room while I get my chemo, "just in case" - just in case what?! Oh my gosh, what possible reaction could I have to these drugs where they wouldn't want my kids to be in the room?! I of course totally understood as I wouldn't want my kids to get traumatized should they witness their mommy have some kind of serious reaction. I got really scared. As my husband and kids left the room, I braced myself. For what - I had no idea.

I should mention that I never sat my kids down to tell them about my breast cancer. They were so young and I wasn't sure how much of it they would even comprehend at their ages. At this point, Maddy didn't even know he was going to his clinic because he had cancer too. There was no real easy way to explain it at the time, so I didn't. All my kids knew was that their mommy was getting medicine that made her hair fall out. Rather than scare them with any more details, I just left it at that.

As I prepared for my second cycle, I thought about my kids and my husband in the other room, and I thought about how much I loved them. I took a deep breath as the nurse administered the first of two chemo drugs. As part of the precautions they were taking, the nurse would stay in the room with me for the first twenty minutes. I remember her asking me, perhaps every five minutes, "How do you feel?" Every time I was thankful to say that I was feeling okay and doing good. As the drugs slowly traveled through the IV and into me, I sat there keenly aware of my body, anticipating, waiting, just waiting, for something to happen and praying that nothing would. After twenty minutes of nothing eventful, the nurse left the room, but frequently checked in on how I was doing. She followed the same drill with the second chemo infusion. They were definitely keeping a close eye on me. Feeling at ease to leave me there to finish up the treatment, Brad took the kids home. By this time, it felt safe to say that the "rechallenge" of the drugs was successful, at least as far as the infusions went. It was the days that followed that were going to be the true test.

Chapter Sixty-Three

By the time I got home, I was pretty exhausted having been at the clinic for the whole afternoon. I spent the rest of that evening feeling a bit apprehensive as I wondered whether there would be some kind of delayed reaction to the chemo. The allergic reaction from the first cycle appeared mostly on my hands. It wasn't itchy, but it looked pretty bad. By this time, although the rash had subsided a bit, my hands still looked quiet red and raw. With the first cycle, the rashes didn't appear until about five days after the infusion. I was curious whether it would be the same with this cycle, or whether it would take longer to appear as they performed a much slower infusion, or whether it would even happen at all. Even though the actual infusions went well with no adverse reactions, I was still on high alert and very aware of any response my body may have to this cycle.

The next afternoon, I got my Neulasta shot. By that evening, I started getting that metallic taste again - just a hint of it, but enough to know that I wouldn't be eating very much for the next week. So far, no rashes.

On Saturday, the queasiness was back and my body just felt out of sorts. I couldn't eat very much because everything tasted awful. I am not kidding when I say that everything literally tasted like paper. When I ran my tongue across my teeth, it just felt dry and icky. I basically had to force myself to eat some food. One of the things I did, which may have been a defense mechanism for me, was stay away from the foods that I really liked. I didn't want to taint the flavor of those foods by eating them while I was on chemo. Even today, there are some foods that I won't eat, or restaurants I won't go into because it reminds me of chemo and that awful taste in my mouth. For example, there was this diner that we went to where I ordered an omelet - oh man, I can still remember the nasty taste and doing my best to get it down. Needless to say, I will probably never eat at that diner again. While I was feeling queasy, I never even tried to eat any of my

favorite foods. In order to protect my love of them, I simply
avoided them until my taste buds recovered.

I also decided not to take any more of the anti-nausea medication.
When I took the one pill back during my first cycle, I was
desperate for it as the nausea was quite severe that particular day.
It didn't really make the nausea go away completely, but it did
relieve it somewhat. Although it subsided, there was still an
overall queasiness I felt throughout the day. I was able to tolerate
this queasiness and so, for the rest of my treatment, I made the
decision to just deal with it. I know some people would think
that's crazy. It's just that in my mind, I was already on all of these
drugs, I didn't want t to have to take any more drugs. Should I feel
it necessary, I knew it was available, but as long as I could manage
the nausea, I wasn't going to take any more medication.

As I mentioned, I had been feeling out of sorts all day that
Saturday and by early evening, I was down for the count. I guess
this was the fatigue they were talking about. I found myself just
overwhelmed with exhaustion. My entire body felt like it had run
a marathon and yet, I didn't do much of anything all day. I was
nauseous, and tired, and just plain wiped out. I wasn't sure
whether I had a head-ache or not, but my head felt heavy, and
foggy, and lightheaded all at the same time. To say that I felt
crummy would not do it justice. It was unlike anything I had ever
felt before. I didn't like this one bit. This made my first cycle
seem like a piece of cake in comparison.

By the way, in case you may have forgotten, in the midst of all of
this, I still had to give Maddox his medicine. Weak from my own
treatment, I would muster all the energy I had so that I could
prepare Maddy's chemo. I don't know how, but I managed to get it
done. It still boggled my mind that my son and I were getting
chemo at the same time. It all seemed too surreal and quite
frankly, really fucked up.

During my treatment, on some of the worst days, I know Brad did
his part to take care of Maddox's medicine. When I had it in me to
summon even the slightest bit of energy, I made myself get up and

do it. As much as possible, I wasn't going to let my condition get in the way of performing this important responsibility.

Later that night, as I lay on the couch, I felt as if I was in a daze. Thankfully, my kids seemed unaware of my mental and physical state as they played all around me. I just kept telling them that Mommy was taking a rest. I think Brad was in the kitchen getting dinner ready. It took every ounce of effort to answer any questions the kids asked me. I was there, but I wasn't. By that point, it took even more effort to get up and eat some sort of dinner. All I wanted was to lie down and go to bed so that I could be done with this day. I went to bed that night hoping for some kind of relief. It was in sleep that I got my escape. While I slept, I didn't feel anything. That was truly my saving grace.

Chapter Sixty-Four

I knew that I made the right decision to choose Thursdays to start the chemo cycles so that I not only had the weekend to be at home to rest, but also so that my husband would be home to pick up the slack. The other choice would have been to start the chemo on Mondays. Had I chosen that, there was no way I would have been able to bring my kids to school and pick them up, much less take care of them while I was basically out of commission. This second cycle was kicking me in the butt. It seemed to be toughest right around the weekend so I was thankful it happened on the days that I had my husband home. I was also extremely thankful to have had my mother-in-law, Cathie come stay with us for several days. She stayed about a week at a time during the most difficult days of my chemo so that she could lend us a hand. This woman was my hero. She watched over the kids. She cooked. She cleaned. She even did our laundry. I honestly don't know how we would have handled all of this without her. She did the same thing during those early months when Maddy was diagnosed, coming to help us take care of everything else so that Brad and I could take care of Maddy. Now she was doing it again, this time so that I could take care of me.

At some point, after hearing the news of my breast cancer diagnosis, Sheryl, one of the directors from Merricat's, the kids' preschool, called me to express her support. In fact, both Linda and Mimi, the other directors from Merricat's, also e-mailed right away, writing me beautiful messages. In the weeks during my treatment, these ladies, just like many of our wonderful friends, sent our family meal after meal realizing that planning what to make for dinner was probably the last thing I wanted to do. Some days, Linda would call and ask what we wanted for dinner that night, and other times, the buzzer would just ring and the doorman would tell us that food was on its way up. Several times, I politely declined Linda's offers as I really didn't want to impose, but she never took no for an answer. For that, I was humbly grateful. These meals were more than welcome, especially on the days when I had no energy to cook, much less grocery shop.

When I was on the phone with Sheryl, she confided in me that she also went through chemo and is a breast cancer survivor. It felt good and reassuring to talk to someone that has been through it and could relate. Sheryl later even let me borrow some of her wigs and head scarves. After bonding over this, she asked whether we would be interested in putting Danika in school full-time. Maddox was already doing full days at school. My first reaction was a bit of surprise because we had signed Danika up for just half days. I loved the idea of Danika going to school full days, but then I thought about how much we'd have to pay - it was after all, private school. With hesitation, I began to inquire about what the fees would be, but I barely got the words out when Sheryl said for us not to worry about it, and that Danika would be placed in the full-time curriculum at no extra cost to us. I was in shock. My heart must have skipped a beat. Oh my goodness. Were they for real? This school had already done so much to support us while Maddy was in treatment, now there they were once again being so giving and thoughtful. As if the meals weren't enough, another Godsend was this amazing gift we got from Merricat's. I was moved to tears. As I humbly accepted this incredibly generous offer, I couldn't even begin to describe the gratitude and love I felt for these wonderful people. Having both of my kids in school full days would give me more time to rest and recuperate while I was on chemo, and I knew in my heart, that that's exactly why they did it. They wanted to do whatever they could to support our family during another difficult situation. It was a true gesture of love.

There are just some kind, decent, and truly good human beings in this world. Our friends at Merricat's Castle School are absolutely among them. For the true generosity and love they have shown our family, this school and the amazing women that run it, will always hold a special place in our hearts. To say that it was a tremendous help to have the extra time to myself to rest and recover from chemo would be not be enough. As I continued with my treatment, I would realize just how much I needed it. In the throes of chemo, it would be my salvation.

Chapter Sixty-Five

Sunday morning arrived and with it came all the fatigue and queasiness from the day before. I peeled myself out of bed just to wash up, brush my teeth, and change. Then I went right back to bed. I'm not kidding. Hey, at least I put on a change of clothes. That was something. Cathie arrived just in time that weekend while I was experiencing the worst of the side effects. I couldn't believe it was possible, but I felt even more tired than I did the day before. To top it off, I was starting to get some joint pain on my neck and shoulders. I was told to expect this side effect from the Neulasta. So in addition to the fatigue, I was now having aches and pains. All I remember was that I must have spent the entire day in my room, in bed, getting up only to get an occasional drink or cracker. It felt like I was hanging on by a thread. I barely had it in me to prepare Maddy's medicine so Brad took care of Maddy's chemo that day. I knew the kids were in good hands with their grandma and their dad so I allowed myself to just hibernate. I was in a stupor. It even hurt to have the TV on. Not even the ridiculous drama of the *Housewives* shows could distract me from my extreme discomfort and tiredness. I was probably in and out of naps all day which did little to make me feel any better. The nurse told me that the upswing usually started on Mondays. Oh, how I begged for Monday.

This "upswing" came very slowly. I still was not myself Monday morning. My body just felt drained. Thank goodness Cathie was there to take the kids to school and pick them up. I looked awful and I felt awful. I ate what I could and took it easy for most of the day. I have to say that it wasn't so much the queasiness that prevented me from eating, it was that horribly dry metal taste in my mouth. I would be hungry and crave something and attempt to eat it, but it would taste just disgusting. It felt like my tongue was rubbing against sand paper. It was during this time of the chemo cycle that I probably lost a lot of weight. Between not getting much sustenance and the fatigue, my body had very little get-up-and-go to do much of anything.

I would say that Monday was a bust. It was on Tuesday that I started to feel a little bit better - physically. Emotionally - well, that was a different story. I think when I was in discomfort, all I could focus on was the physical exhaustion. I was too tired to feel or concentrate on anything else. Ironically, it was as my body was starting to recover from the chemo, that I began to get depressed. I started to really process what was happening to me. I thought of being in my room all day that previous Sunday while I heard my kids playing in the living room. I felt sad that I couldn't be a part of all the laughter and activity. It felt like life was going on as usual all around me, and there I was, forced by my condition to be an outsider in my own home. It was a very lonely feeling. I suppose I could have rested on the couch to be nearer to my family like I did that Saturday, but by Sunday, I just didn't have it in me. I was too weak and pathetic. I absolutely did not want my kids to see me, their mommy like that. On the worst days when it felt like everything hurt, it was for the best that I just be left alone.

As my body slowly felt the upswing that Tuesday, my emotions took a turn in the opposite direction. I fell deeper into my depression. This would be one of those moments that I let myself wallow in my situation. Perhaps it was because this round of chemo really hit me hard. Prior to this, I'd like to think I was doing a pretty good job keeping my chin up. At least I thought so. On this day, I felt sorry for myself and boy did I go for it. That afternoon, I sat in the dining room nibbling on some food just staring off into nothing, letting this feeling of hopelessness build inside me. I felt lost. Cathie was at the table, sitting across from me, playing some game on the I-Pad. It was quiet except for the many loud thoughts in my mind. I sat there wearing a cap to cover my bald head and I thought about what I looked like. I thought about what people think when they see someone wearing a cap or scarf over their obviously bald head, because it's what I would think. Cancer. I could picture the sadness and more unbearable, the pity on their faces as they knew that person must be getting chemo. I thought, "Oh my gosh, that's what I look like. That's me. I was the cancer patient." It started slowly at first, with the tears welling up in my eyes, and then all at once, all of the emotion I was feeling that was bubbling inside me, finally burst. I let it all out. The schools' winter break was approaching right around this time and I heard many friends and other moms talk about the vacations they were getting ready to take. Many of them talked about taking their kids to Disney World or some other exciting destination. I found myself feeling so achingly jealous. I thought about how wonderful it must be to plan all of these amazing trips for the kids' winter vacation. Then I thought about us. With Maddox and I both in treatment, we were not making any of those plans. I couldn't stop crying as I shared all of these emotions and thoughts with Cathie. She came over and put her arms around me and allowed me to vent, to be sad, to be bitter, to be angry, to be whatever I needed to be. I felt emotionally broken as I wept like a child and said, "When are we going to go on these vacations? When are we going to plan those trips? Why can't our family be normal? Why is this happening to us?" There were no simple answers to those questions. All I remember was Cathie telling me over and over again, "You will go on vacations. You will." I was hearing her, but in that moment, I had a hard time believing it. It all just seemed so far away, so distant. Struggling to recover from this round of chemo, I had a hard time thinking beyond that point. For a few minutes, I gave myself over to my emotions and just cried. Eventually, I had had enough of this tantrum. I had my mini meltdown and it was time to get myself together. Just like that, I turned that part of me that wanted to wallow - off.

Adapt and Overcome. That was our family's motto during my son's treatment, and now, they would continue to be the words that guide me through my own treatment.

Chapter Sixty-Six

That was a rough week, much more so than the first cycle. This second round sure took a toll on me. Despite the emotional set backs, there were some good things to focus on. As far as the rashes were concerned, I did notice just a touch of it appear on my hands on that Tuesday, but it was no where near what it looked like with the first cycle. Giving me a slower infusion appeared to have worked, and it seemed that I could safely say that I had passed that "rechallenge." I was also extremely relieved that I had no bladder irritation. I was very, very grateful for that. Giving me that extra infusion of saline did the trick. Although the nausea was unpleasant, it was manageable, and I was able to stay off the anti-nausea medication. By midweek I was tired, but nothing like I had experienced over the weekend. By the following Saturday, my taste buds were back to normal.

As I entered into my good week, the aches from the joint pain were gone and there was a definite difference in the way my whole body felt. It sort of felt like it was regaining back its senses. Like an unwanted guest who had overstayed it's welcome, that second round of chemo was finally getting out of my system. My upswing was set in motion and I was so ready for it. I would have about a week and a half of feeling "normal" before Round 3.

I took full advantage of this time and did all the things I needed to get done. I did the laundry, I did housekeeping, I did the food shopping - basically, all the essential activities were taken care of before my next cycle. While that was all well and good, one of the things I looked forward to the most during this week and a half break was that I got to EAT! It was a beautiful thing. I relished and really appreciated everything I ate. Screw diets! Screw the calories! I was going to indulge and I did. I even remember randomly buying a whole chocolate mouse cake one day. I really did. It was pure joy biting into something that tasted like it was supposed to taste. The joy of a good meal was my simple pleasure. It is amazing how much I have come to appreciate these ordinary things. Even the simple act of just walking out the door, feeling the sun on my face, and feeling the strength in my body, was both amazing and humbling because these are things we can often and easily take for granted. I remember one beautiful day walking to pick up the kids from school, I stopped where I was, took a moment, looked around at the activity all around me, took it all in, and just simply felt grateful to be out and about, grateful to be active, so grateful that my body felt good.

I even made it to the gym every day that week. I did find it interesting, but not that surprising how people looked at me at the gym. Obviously I would not want to wear my wigs working out so I wore my cap. Prior to being diagnosed with breast cancer, I'm proud to say that I was a regular at the gym. As a regular, there were those of us who went at the same time. Although we never really spoke, we knew our faces. The first time I went to the gym with my cap on, I felt very self-conscious. I acted like nothing was different, but inside I didn't want anyone to notice me. I just wanted to get my sixty minutes in and get the heck out of dodge.

Upon seeing me, some of the "regulars" did the whole stare, then quickly look away bit. It was so painfully obvious. Those who did take a moment to look, had to look twice as if they couldn't believe their eyes. For a split second, they didn't recognize me and then, I could see it register in their faces. I would be like, "Yep, you guessed it. Cancer patient comin' through." These people would politely smile at me, but it wasn't the usual, typical smile of the casual pleasantries one would exchange at the gym. Their smiles had a hint of the, "I'm so sorry" look. That was the worst. Of course, this may have all been my imagination. But more likely than not, I saw what I saw for what it was - the honest reaction of people being face to face with cancer.

I got a similar response whenever I was in the laundry room. I saw the same looks of concern and polite smiles. I guess I should have milked this sympathy for all it was worth so that they would have let me get to the washing machines first without waiting - ha! For all I know, some of them may have done just that. On one particular occasion, one of the building staff guys that I was friendly with, happened to be in the laundry room when he noticed me. Within seconds, I saw the transformation on his face as his expression went from pleasant, to a bit of confusion, then shock, to worry. That was the typical reaction I got from people who knew me when they saw me for the first time in my "cancer cap." He came over to me and asked me how I was doing. I smiled and told him that I was doing well. With a look of worry, he quickly replied back, "Are you sure?" Apparently he did not believe me. I told him that yes, I was sure, hoping to put an end to this conversation, and it did. I had almost the same exact conversation with other staff members that I encountered in the building whenever I wasn't wearing one of my wigs. I'm pretty sure they all had a good idea what was going on, but I was not interested in discussing it with any of them. Thankfully nobody pressed the issue, and they let me go on about my business. It was nice that they cared, but I appreciated even more, for the most part, that they respected my privacy. There were very few people that knew what I was going through and I wanted to keep it that way.

With my energy at a good level, I was also able to bring Maddox and Danika to school and pick them up. I was able to play with them and fully enjoy my kids. That was the real gift. It was a great feeling to have this routine back. I needed it. This was my time of bliss. Those were precious days to me because I knew it wouldn't be long before my next chemo infusion.

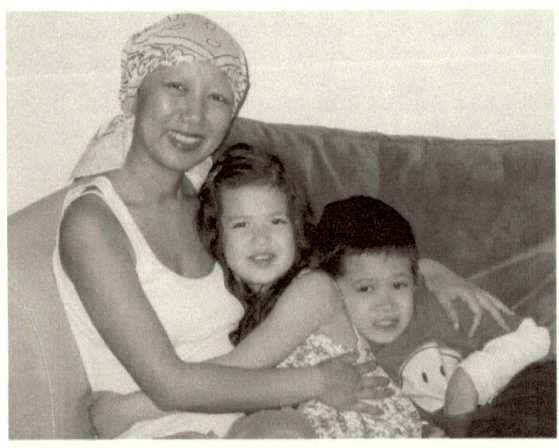

Chapter Sixty-Seven

With these first two cycles under my belt, I now had a sense of what to expect and when. I knew that it was the first week and a half after the infusion that I would basically be useless. In this boxing match, I knew the major hits would come on that first weekend - the nausea, the joint pain, the metallic mouth - those were the right hooks and upper cuts. Based on the second cycle, I knew that the extreme fatigue would be the knock-out punch - literally.

By the time I prepared for my third round of chemo, I certainly did not have the same bravado I had when I started my first cycle. Back then I stupidly thought it wouldn't be that bad. I was confident in that thought. Well, chemo certainly put me in my place. I keep making these boxing references because that's the closest thing to which I could equate this experience. It's like a rookie getting in the ring with the heavy weight champion of the world. Who does that?! At first, you get that first punch, but are strong enough and dare I say, cocky enough, to shake it off. Then as the hits keep coming, you realize you are no match for this monster. Eventually, you are down for the count, with no strength or even desire to get up. You just beg for the ding of that bell so that you know that it's over. As difficult as it was getting chemo treatment, I knew that it was a necessary evil. Ultimately, my opponent became my ally in this fight against the true enemy - cancer.

The third round was basically a carbon copy of the second cycle, with one *major* difference - the fatigue. All the usual suspects assaulted my body yet again, but man oh man, the fatigue was ruthless. I knew that it would be cumulative with each cycle, but this was no joke. A friend of mine who had also done chemo for breast cancer described it perfectly. She said that it felt like you had the body of a ninety year old lady. She was so right.

In this third cycle, I felt incredibly worn down not only physically, but also mentally. I know I have had some emotional breakdowns during this whole experience, how could I not? This time, I felt even more defeated. I would stare at myself in the mirror and what I saw was not me. My face was pale and the skin around my eyes looked sunken and dark. I had no eyelashes to speak of, and I could literally count the number of hairs on my eyebrows. There may have been like five or six of them bravely hanging on. Then there were my fingernails. The chemo discolors them and makes them dark and black. The rashes on my hands were faded, but the scars from them were still there. Damn, I looked like a sick person. I felt so ugly, so sad, so deflated. This third round of chemo was a bitch.

My body felt so frail. I remember one night, laying in bed, with Brad's arm around me, feeling particularly drained beyond all comprehension, when I simply said to him, "I don't think I can do this." And I really meant it. I didn't think I could go on with the chemo. I flashed back once again to that horrific moment when Maddy was at the hospital and the nurses kept poking and sticking him with needles, trying to find his veins He didn't have his port in place yet, so the nurses had to access him through his arm. I remember Brad holding Maddy down while he wriggled and screamed in pain and fear. It tore my heart to pieces. I wanted to scream at the nurses to stop. I wanted all of it to just stop. I stood there watching my son crying and all I heard was him yelling over and over again, "All done! All done!" I painfully thought of that day as I was going through my chemo hell and like my son, in my head, I too was screaming, "All done! All done!"

Even though I knew that I only had one more chemo cycle left, it was so bad, that I not only didn't think I could do it, I didn't want to do it anymore. Brad just held me closer and said, "Please, just think of me and the kids." Those words shot straight to my heart. I DID think of him and the kids. I thought about them *all* the time. I thought about graduations, I thought about helping Danika pick out her wedding dress, I thought about that special dance with my son on his wedding day, I thought about growing old with my husband, and I thought about everything in between, and when I thought about all of those things, I prayed, oh how I begged, with *everything* I had in me, "Please God, please, *please* let me live.

Please God, let me survive this. Please let me be there for my family to do all of those wonderful things." I tried to control these emotions all night so when I finally let it out, it was a deep, and rushed, and heavy cry, the kind of cry when it feels like you can't catch your breath. Once again, I was reduced to a puddle of tears. Brad just held me tighter, but I would not be comforted that night. I wanted to be brave. I wanted to be strong. I willed myself not to give up, but this round of chemo brought me to my knees. It breaks your spirit. Beaten down, all I could do in that moment was submit to these emotions and hope that the last cycle of chemo didn't kill me. For the first time, I had no fight left in me. In the quiet of the night, with so many thoughts going through my head, I just let the tears fall onto my already soaked pillow.

Chapter Sixty-Eight

The following days just sort of blended together. I was still in a funk, but I kept it to myself. I knew that I was more than half way through my chemo treatment, but it was a victory I couldn't celebrate. I felt like an emotional yo-yo. It was during those toughest weeks of the chemo cycle that I would go through such incredible lows when my emotions would get the best of me. Chemo makes you go to a dark place. Some days I honestly felt like I wasn't going to find my way out of it. But somehow, even at my lowest of lows, when it felt like I had no fight left in me, I never lost my resolve. It may have been beaten and bruised quite a bit, but incredibly, it was still there, and it was just enough to keep me going. Stand up and fight! It was the love of my family and my children that gave me the determination to press on. In them, I found the light in each new day. I was going to get through this. I would do it for my beautiful children. I would do it for my husband. I would do it for me.

It was with this mindset that I approached my fourth and final cycle of chemo. I knew what I was getting into and all I kept saying to myself was, "It's the last one, Geri. It's the last one." I knew that the finish line was in my sights. At my check-up before the infusions, the doctor congratulated me and said, "Last one!" In my mind I knew all too well that I still had to go through a bit of hell to be really done with it. So while I wasn't quite ready to do a dance or anything, it did feel damn good to hear her say it.

Sitting in the treatment room, watching the nurse prepare the needle, I looked at my arms and saw the scars of all the places they poked me. They never put the needle in the same place so for me, each scar represented each cycle of chemo. They would be my battle scars, a proud reminder that even in my weakest moments, I found the strength to lift myself up and finish what I started. Some hours later, the final round of chemo infusions were done. As I left the treatment room for the last time, I exhaled and did not look back. There were no surprises during the three weeks of that last cycle. Yes, it was brutal. Yes, it beat me down. But more importantly, hell YES, it was the last one! The final cycle was certainly no picnic to say the least, but I was finally done. I did it. Praise the Lord!

Chapter Sixty-Nine

Radiation

I had about a month break before I would begin radiation. From everything I've heard - after chemo, radiation would be no sweat. Before the actual radiation began, they had me come in to take measurements of the areas to pinpoint, as well as to do a practice run. They would perform radiation and target the area where I had my lumpectomy, doing their best to avoid, as much as possible, hitting other major organs, like my lungs and heart. I obviously was not comforted by these thoughts. I was told that these were the risks with radiation. Of course I was scared, but I had no choice. It was just another part of my treatment, an essential part to keep me cancer-free. In the trial run, they were able to use a technique on me where I would take a deep breath and hold it in during the radiation. The zap would take anywhere from twenty to thirty seconds. The deep breath pulls the other organs away from the target area. This strategy allows the radiologists to focus on the main area, while decreasing the risk of hitting the lungs and heart. The radiologists were satisfied with this method, and so I would get 16 sessions of radiation therapy, one session per day, every day, not including the weekends, for the next 4 weeks.

The main side effect of radiation is fatigue. Great. There's that "F" word again. I was just starting to bounce back from the chemo, only to be worn down again by radiation. Some of the technicians said that the fatigue comes mostly from having to come everyday, rather than the actual radiation itself. Whatever. It made no difference to me at that point. Tired was tired. Nevertheless, I was more than grateful that that was the only side effect to be expected. I wouldn't have called getting zapped every day a piece of cake, but it was a hell of a lot better than getting chemo.

The radiation itself was rather simple. There was some minor discomfort laying on the table, but overall, once I was in there and set up on the table, it went fairly quickly. It was the waiting to get in the room that was actually the most tedious. Some days, I would be in the sitting area waiting for three hours just to get zapped for thirty seconds.

The waiting room was awful. I was always relieved when I finally heard my name called to go in, even if I didn't have a very long wait. Unlike the Evelyn H. Lauder Breast Center that only dealt with breast cancer patients, the waiting room to get radiation at Sloan Kettering was filled with all varieties of cancer patients, a virtual smorgasbord. I found that there were basically two types of people in the waiting room. There were the people that wanted to share all the details of their cancer experience, and then there were the people that wanted them to just keep their traps shut. It's not too difficult to guess which category I came in. I don't want to sound insensitive, but I really didn't want to hear about this person's tumor or that person's complications. I certainly did not want to hear people comparing notes, "Well this happened to me. What happened to you?" What I really wanted was to scream, "Shut the fuck up! You are freaking me out!" I wanted to run far away from these people and their graphic conversations. I understand that for many people, it helps to talk about and share their experiences, but I was plenty scared enough for myself. I sure as hell didn't want to include other people's fears with my own. There were some days that I would literally have to get up and take a random walk down the hallway just so that I didn't have to listen to some person's horror stories. Talk about wanting some ear-muffs. Get me outta here! Cancer is not pretty. Hearing other people's account of it was torture. Yes, I know. Here I am, sharing my cancer story and all the details of it, but the major difference is, you are *choosing* to read it. At the waiting room, I sometimes did not have a choice but to sit there and hear stories that scared the hell out of me. All I wanted was just to keep to myself and sit there reading my magazine, in peace and quite, until my name was called. Was that so much to ask??? Each day I did my best to find a quiet corner and prayed that whoever sat next to me would value privacy as much as I did.

While I am on this rant, the other thing that I never understood when I told people that I had breast cancer, was how some of them would immediately tell me about the people they knew that died of cancer. Some of them would even tell me about the people they knew who had died specifically from breast cancer. They would say something to the effect of, "Well you know, my mother died of breast cancer." It would be either that or they would say it was their aunt, their grandma, or their co-worker. My question is this: "Why in the hell would you tell a breast cancer patient about someone dying of breast cancer?!!!" It really baffled me. How was I supposed to respond or react to a comment like that? "Gee, um, thanks for sharing???" All I could do was sit there dumbfounded. I know some of these people were my family and friends that I love, but really??? It was ludicrous to me. There has to be some sensitivity to the situation where they should have realized that I obviously would not be comforted by those comments. Duh! My greatest fear was to die from this disease. Why would anyone, with any common sense, think that it's okay to say that to me. Yes, I know it was probably said with caring intentions, but trust me, that is one of the worst things you can say to a cancer patient.

Attention! Cancer patients sure as hell don't want to hear about other people that are dead because of the very thing they are fighting. To those of you who said stuff like that to me, I forgive you, but honestly, what an incredibly inappropriate thing to say.

Take note people. We want to hear about people in remission, we want to hear about Survivors, we want to hear about people that are CURED! Comprende!!! Good. Now you know better. Thank you for listening. Whew, that felt good to get that out.

Chapter Seventy

Having to get radiation for 16 sessions was kind of depressing. Every day, sometimes for hours at a time, I'd sit there surrounded by all of these sick people, myself included. Some of them looked like they were in really bad shape. Having to witness that and be there every day, for almost four weeks, really effects you. It certainly got to me. It made me sad not just for myself, but for all those people fighting their own battles. It's like when I took Maddy to his Clinic visits - I would sit there and sometimes, I would just quietly observe the other families with their children. You just a feel a heaviness in your heart. You feel the weight of all their concerns and fears because they are yours too. Every day for sixteen days, sitting there with those people waiting to get radiation, it is easy to let depression take hold of you. For all the pain and suffering that going through cancer treatment causes, sometimes the hardest thing to bear is the overwhelming sadness.

Chapter Seventy-One

About half way through radiation treatment, I started to experience some back pain. At the time, I wasn't too concerned as I attributed it to probably laying on that table every day. The last time I remembered having that back pain was when I was walking back and forth from home to be with Maddox when he was at the hospital, which was a little over a mile each way. Once I got good walking shoes, the back pain went away. I figured this time around, it was all the laying on the table, and all the walking I was doing to and from the radiation clinic, that was causing the back pain. On a couple of occasions, I mentioned the back pain to the radiologist. The first time we talked about it, she discussed possibly getting an MRI to investigate the back pain. I was immediately struck with fear. I never thought I would have to get an MRI! I honestly thought that the back pain was no big deal. I didn't want to get an MRI. More to the point, I was terrified of what the MRI would find. I couldn't even speak it. So each time the radiologist mentioned it, I would tell her about the back pain I had when I was doing a lot of walking to visit my son when he was at the hospital, and that it eventually went away once I got better shoes. I also talked about how laying on that table was a possible cause of the back pain. I tried to find any reason I could in order to avoid getting that MRI. I wanted to convince her that I thought the back pain would resolve itself on its own once the radiation treatment was done.

Somehow I managed to have her hold off, but it didn't provide me with much relief as deep down I knew it was probably best to have gotten the MRI. I knew it would have been the smart thing to do. The whole notion that it is far better to catch something early - if there was something to catch - was constantly on my mind. But I was just so scared. I wanted to believe that it was nothing. I didn't think I could take another blow. I just had to believe that it was all harmless. As the weeks passed and the back pain persisted, I grew more and more anxious.

At a follow-up exam with my oncologist, I reluctantly told her about the back pain. When she too suggested getting an MRI, I could not hold it off any longer. I guess when you're a cancer patient, any kind of pain is a cause for concern. Then the doctor said what I dreaded and feared the most, but would not let myself think or say out loud. She said very matter-of-factly, "Let's get the MRI to make sure that the cancer did not spread." Oh my God, oh my God, oh my God. My no big deal back pain, was now a huge deal. I wanted to cry. I knew I had to be brave and get the MRI done. I had to do it because not knowing one way or the other was torture. I kept my composure, but inside I was trembling with terror. I couldn't concentrate on anything else she was saying. All I kept thinking over and over was, "Please don't let it be cancer. Please don't let it be cancer." I just finished fucking chemo for fuck's sake! I went home in a daze wrapped in nothing but fear.

My husband was there when I got home and as soon as I saw him, I told him that I needed him. I cried as I told him that I had to get an MRI. I could barely get the words out to explain why the doctor wanted me to get it done. I felt so powerless. When was I going to stop fearing for my life???! When was I going to stop feeling so damn scared???! When the hell was I going to stop crying???! I was so over this. Brad held me and did his best to comfort me. He was very calm about it. One of us had to keep it together. That job whether he wanted it or not, fell on him. I know it must have been a hell of a job, but he did it. Sometimes, I wondered whether he was just very practical and rational about everything, and other times I wondered how much strength it must have taken for him not to break down with me. Through everything we've been through, Brad has shown so much grace under fire. I wish the same could be said for me. Too many times I let my emotions get the best of me. This time would be no different. I was really worried. It would near impossible to think of anything else until I got those MRI results.

Chapter Seventy-Two

The MRI

As you can imagine, I scheduled the MRI as soon as I could get it. After avoiding it for so long, now I just wanted it over and done with as quickly as possible. The MRI is a very intimidating process. It's just you in that narrow tube. You can't move and you certainly can't have anyone hold your hand through it. You basically just lie there counting the minutes until they let you out, praying that you don't have to hit the panic button. On the day of the MRI, I did my best to stay calm. I heard some people recommend taking a Xanax before the procedure. I didn't want to do that. I've had enough of drugs. My husband came with me to the appointment, but I knew he couldn't be in the room with me during the MRI. They happened to be running late that day and I thought, "Oh great, more time to sit here and let my nerves get the best of me." I found myself taking lots of deep breaths to calm my mind and not think about being in that contraption. I was afraid I was going to hyperventilate with all of those deep breaths! When they finally called me in, I was just on the very edge of full on freak out mode. This was it.

My body and hands were shaking like a leaf as I got undressed and put on that medical gown. When I walked in the room, I avoided taking a good look at the machine. Then they told me I was going to be in there for about 45 minutes. Son a bitch! Forty five minutes! That sounded like an eternity. I took several more calming breaths as they laid me on the table, but calm I wasn't. The technician gave me the button and explained that I can press it at anytime should I want to get out. I wasn't even in there yet and I was like, "Can I press it now?" The technician gave me ear plugs and I felt my hands trembling as I put them on. She finished setting me up and soon, as I lay there with my heart beating out of my chest, I felt the table begin to move. I closed my eyes. As I got further inside, I sensed the brightness from the room begin to fade. I was in. More deep breaths.

Once the technician started, all I heard was this very loud "boing" sound over and over again. Boing! Boing! Boing! It was incredibly loud. I guess that's what the ear plugs were for. In a muffled voice, I heard her ask me ask me every few minutes how I was doing. I wanted to say, "Quit talking to me and just get on with it!" Instead I just replied that I was okay, but boy, I sure had a very firm grip on that button, prepared to press it if I had to. More than a couple of times, I allowed myself to peek out, but always quickly shut my eyes when all I saw was this machine surrounding me in the darkness.

I have to say that what helped me get through this process were my kids. As I prepared for the MRI, I had this idea and I went with it. During the MRI, with my eyes closed, I had a running slide show of the many pictures I've taken of my kids. In my mind, I looked at baby pictures, birthday pictures, holiday pictures, every picture I could remember, and I looped them over and over again. All I saw were Maddox's and Danika's beautiful faces and their incredible smiles. In my head, I replayed videos of my kids dancing or singing, and with that, I was able to transport myself back to those precious moments, allowing myself to escape the reality of where I really was. It worked. The more I lost myself in those delightful images, the looser my grip was on that button. My amazing kids got me through it.

After what felt like an eternity, the technician gave me the five minute mark. As soon as I felt the conveyor belt move and felt the light of the room shining back on me, I opened my eyes and breathed a sigh of relief. It was over. I did it. As I prepared to leave, I tried to read the technician's face to see whether it gave any indication of the results, but nothing. She just told me that my doctor would call probably the next day with the report. With that, I couldn't get out of there quick enough.

After I left, I did my best to focus on other things. The next day, I practically ran for the phone every time it rang. Finally, I saw my doctor's caller ID. I quickly answered it. My heart was racing as I gripped the phone to my ear, "Hello." My doctor simply said, "Hi Geri, your MRI is clear. It's not cancer." With those powerful words, I nearly dropped to the ground in pure, absolute, and overwhelming relief. I thanked her, got off the phone, and said out loud with all the conviction that I felt, "Oh thank you Lord God in Heaven!!! Thank you!!!" I was emotionally drained by this whole experience, but so incredibly grateful for the outcome. After that, I was able to continue my radiation treatment with more confidence and way less drama!

Chapter Seventy-Three

On one of the days I had radiation, I noticed a group of people in the waiting room with "Congratulations" signs and colorful balloons. I figured that they were the friends and family of someone getting radiation. It was obvious that it was that person's last day of treatment. When the woman came out, there was boisterous clapping, followed by hugs and cheers all around. As I observed this festive scene in front of me, I was moved by all of this show of support and encouragement. Whoever thought a celebratory mood could take over this usually somber sitting room, but in that moment, it did. I must admit that I felt a little jealous, not only because she was done with radiation, but because I knew I probably wouldn't have a cheering crowd greet me with hugs, kisses, and balloons when I was done. It's mostly my fault because as private as I was, I didn't tell many, if any of my friends, about my radiation schedule, and as much as I love my husband, I wasn't sure it was something he would think to coordinate. Despite this momentary jealousy, watching this woman's family and friends congratulate her, I smiled as did many others in the room. I can't speak for everyone, but it sure lifted me up. I was genuinely happy for her because I knew it must have been a long road to get there. It was a cause for celebration. There was a sense of hope in the air and it felt good. I thought to myself, only a few more sessions and I too can kiss this place good bye.

It wasn't long after that day that I had my last radiation treatment, and although there was little pomp and circumstance to commemorate the day, it felt good all the same. At home later that afternoon, I did get a delivery of a beautiful bouquet of flowers from my husband and kids, with a note congratulating me on finishing my treatment, and telling me that they loved me. There may not have been balloons and decorations, but there was a whole lotta love. That was all I needed to honor and celebrate this very significant and special occasion.

Chapter Seventy-Four

As I mentioned earlier, one of the side effects I experienced during my chemo was that one of the drugs made my fingernails turn a dark color. Once I finished my chemo treatment, the dark coloring began to fade and slowly but surely with each passing day, I noticed my nails get lighter and lighter, back to their normal shade. I often found myself looking at my nails, watching the dark color grow out from the tips. Each day, they sort of became markers of my healing process. It reminded me of what I went through during chemo. As I look at them now, several months after completing treatment, the darkness is almost completely grown out and very soon, those last remnants of the chemo's side effects would no longer be there.

I may have healed physically, but emotionally I am still recovering. I would soon learn that dealing with the emotional "fallout" from my experiences would be one of the most difficult challenges I would have to overcome. Sometimes I wonder whether I will ever fully recover mentally and emotionally from everything I've been through with my son's treatment and my own.

Chapter Seventy-Five

Tamoxifen

It was two days after finishing radiation that I began my hormone therapy. This involves taking a pill called tamoxifen every day. Since my pathology showed that I was estrogen positive, taking tamoxifen would suppress the estrogen, which then reduces the risk of breast cancer, and improves survival rates. I was told that this drug may cause pre-menopause, as well as the side effects that come with it, like hot flashes. I thought that is certainly a small price to pay to save my life.

Some time has passed since I began this book. As I write this, I have been on tamoxifen for over a year now. While it is easy enough to pop a pill every day, taking this drug did not come without some challenges, particularly for my marriage. In addition to the occasional hot flashes, I have experienced moodiness and fatigue that hits me at random moments. I guess that shouldn't be surprising since it is hormone therapy. It's like having PMS, only 10 times stronger. I didn't notice it so much when I first started the drug, but in the past recent months, it has certainly made itself known. My husband can attest to that.

I remember one night we had a huge argument. There were certainly raised voices and hurtful comments thrown in both directions. Interestingly enough, I don't remember the specifics of what we were fighting about, but it had something to do with house chores. For some reason, we constantly fight about that silliness, as I think most married couples do. While this was not the first time we have blown up at each other these past months, what I do remember is that this was the first time I had brought up the effects that the tamoxifen was having on me. Sometimes the fatigue just hits me without warning and my body really feels it.

This particular night, I was really wiped out. I was in the kitchen cleaning up and I was annoyed that Brad wasn't helping. It felt like I was doing all the cleaning, all the time and I told him so.

Brad got angry that I was making a big deal out of nothing. He
didn't understand that this drug can sometimes make me really
tired and moody, which then makes me even more sensitive to
things that maybe are not such a big deal. I resented that he
couldn't understand that. Brad said something to the effect that I
was being lazy - he actually used the word, lazy! Well, that set me
off. We really got into it after that. I was extremely offended by
that comment. I certainly was not lazy! As he fully well knows, I
clean that kitchen every night. How dare he say that! I know this
argument may sound ridiculous, but at the heart of it was a very
real issue. I was so angry, I let him have it. I told him how
insensitive he was to what this drug was doing to me. I told him
that sometimes I just don't have the same energy that I used to
have. I yelled and told him that he should have more compassion
that my body was not the same because of everything it went
through with the chemo, and now, because of what it was going
through with the tamoxifen. He knows what chemo did to me and
my body. Of all people, he should have understood. It hurt that I
had to explain this to him. Then naturally, I stormed off. I hated
arguing with my husband, but it felt good to have finally let that all
out.

After we both sort of cooled off, Brad approached me and
apologized. That is one of the many great things about Brad. He
more often than not, will be the first one to make things better. He
told me that he didn't realize what kind of effects the tamoxifen
was having on me. I couldn't fault him for that because up until
that day, I never really told him. Brad has handled a lot, more than
any husband and father should have to deal with. He had to be
strong so many times, first for his son, and then for me. When we
talked, he told me that he thought when I finished my chemo
treatment, that things would go back to "normal." While we were
informed by my doctor of all the possible side effects of the
chemo, we never really went into detail about what the possible
effects might be, with the exception of the hot flashes, from the
tamoxifen. Brad said if he knew all of this ahead of time, he would
have at least been able to prepare himself for my moodiness and
fatigue. We had made up, but were both emotionally exhausted

and saddened that dealing with this was another obstacle we had to overcome.

Even after that talk, I think that Brad sometimes forgets that my body is not the same, or that I take this hormone pill every day. A few days after that blow up, I was with Maddy at one of his check-ups and I got to talking to one of his doctors, Dr. Gary. He knew that I had finished treatment for breast cancer and that I was now on tamoxifen. He asked me how I was doing and I confided in him about what this drug was doing to me - the moodiness, the fatigue, all of that. He was not at all surprised. In fact, he even gave me a knowing look of understanding and told me that he's heard similar experiences from other women that were on that drug. I was so relieved to have talked to him. I felt validation. I wanted to hug him because parts of me thought that maybe it was just me, and that I was being a bitch for no reason. There was a reason! I told him that it was impacting my relationship with Brad. He told me that Brad has to understand that tamoxifen is a drug that influences the hormones and consequently, the emotions. He compared it to when Maddox was on steroids. I would have never thought of it that way. He was like, "Just try to remember what the steroids did to Maddy when he was on it for just a week." Of course I remember! I will never forget it. In addition to the extreme hunger, when Maddox was on steroids, he was very irritable and very, very moody. He was a completely different kid. When Dr. Gary said that, a light bulb went on. To me that was the best way to explain to Brad what I was going through. I was so grateful to Dr. Gary simply for acknowledging it. That night I told Brad about my conversation with Dr. Gary and his reference to when Maddox was on the steroids. He agreed that it made sense. All I can say is that he got it. Halleluiah! Brad finally got it. Now, all he had to do was remember that whenever I got temperamental. Somehow, I knew that was going to be easier said than done.

Chapter Seventy-Six

I wish I didn't have to be on this drug. At times, it can make me so sensitive and yes, probably a moody bitch. Earlier I wrote about how being diagnosed with breast cancer has given me a new outlook on life. That is very true. I appreciate so many things so much more. In addition, I am doing my best not to let the little things get to me. While my husband may disagree, I honestly feel I am making an effort to do that. With my kids, I am great at it. I am so much more patient and understanding with all things related to my kids. I am very proud of that. I have to honestly say that my experience has made me a better mother. As a wife...well, Brad may have a thing or two to say about that.

In recent months, since being on hormone therapy, not "sweating the small stuff " with my husband has not been such an as easy task. Even after our talk, Brad and I have gotten into countless arguments over these so called little things - again probably related to house chores, like whose turn it was to wash the dishes - or we'd fight about his video game addiction. When I'm feeling moody, my annoyance factor hits the Richter scale and these "little things" become huge issues. Meanwhile, Brad would say things like "Relax" or "Let it go" or "What's the big deal?" Man, there is nothing more infuriating than when someone, with as calm as can be an attitude, tells you to "Relax" over and over again, especially when you are already very riled up! Brad knew it would push my buttons and that made it even worse. When we have these flare ups, I wish I didn't have to remind him that it's not me talking, that instead it's me having one of those "tamoxifen" moments. It's easy for him to forget that I take this pill every day. I, on the other hand, am very conscious of it. I know he shouldn't have to remember that every time we fight, but you know what, he really does!

Here's the thing. I am very well aware that in a lot of instances, Brad is probably right. That I should let "it" go, whatever "it" may be at the time. Of course I know that some of the things we fight about are silly and unnecessary, but in the moment they are anything but. In his frustration, Brad says mean and hurtful things, which only adds fuel to the flame. Sometimes I feel like have no control over my emotions, and things just escalate to these knock down drag out fights. It is very scary and very frustrating for me. I wish Brad understood that more. I don't want to be that person. It would be great if I got a heads up whenever I am going to turn into Mr. Hyde so that I can warn Brad to steer clear, but it is not always that simple. These mood swings are very random. It is very easy for my husband to say, "Relax" and "Let it go," but what he doesn't realize is that it is often not so easy to put things into the "proper" perspective when raging hormones are at play. This is what I struggle with the most when those moments hit. Trying to strike a balance between what you know is a "little thing," and what your hormones are doing to make you feel like it's not, is really a battle. I never know which one is going to prevail - the sensible or the irrational. I hate that I don't have more control over it. I hate that it causes a rift between my husband and me.

I have to be on tamoxifen for five years. On my most recent visit with my doctor, she said that research shows taking tamoxifen for ten years to be of even greater benefit to survival rates. Ten years! That's a heck of a lot of tamoxifen. For the sake of my marriage, I have to get a handle on it. I love my husband so I am determined to do just that. I may not always succeed, but I really am trying. Ultimately, despite the "inconveniences" that comes with this drug, I stand by my belief that taking this little pill every day is a very small price to pay to save my life. I know that even though my husband may not like me very much at times, he would agree.

To our family and friends we appeared to be the fun loving couple they're used to, but in reality, it felt like our marriage was in trouble. I guess we put on a great act because no one was the wiser. To me, it seemed like we were fighting more that we were loving. Apparently, Brad thought so too. That week, after our huge blow up, Brad comes home from work and says, "Please don't get mad, but I made a phone call." I looked at him apprehensively and slowly said, "Okay..." It turns out that he made an appointment for us to see a counselor. With that announcement, I didn't feel anger. I felt love. He cared enough about us and our marriage to make the first step towards getting our relationship back on track. He explained that he thought it would be good for us to talk to someone about what we were going through and I agreed. Brad is a good man.

At this point, I should clarify that Brad and I weren't fighting every day. We had and have, many good and loving moments. It's just that lately, when we did fight, they tended to be kind of explosive. I should also add that it's not fair to say that tamoxifen was the source of all of our marital issues. It wasn't. I certainly don't want anyone thinking that I was this emotional freak waiting to erupt at any given moment. I wasn't. Some of the arguments we had were completely valid and not based on these "little things" that were blown out of proportion. There was something more going on between Brad and me. We were not communicating the way we used to. There were often lots of, "he said, she said" issues where he wouldn't remember something I clearly said, and vice versa. That drove us both bananas! It was exhausting and eventually, it began to feel like we were just picking our battles in order to keep the peace in our relationship. I don't know, maybe that is something all marriages go through. I'm sure that other married couples complain of similar things. But perhaps because of what Brad and I have been through, our arguments are coming from a different place. It just seemed that lately, Brad and I were not in tune. We were way out of tune. We were not the "us" that we know and love.

On another one of Maddox's check-ups, I approached one of the social workers we were friendly with, and explained what was going on in my marriage. I felt comfortable reaching out to these people because they knew our history very well and it felt safe to confide in them. I knew there would be no judgment. They could listen with an objective ear, unlike family and friends who would probably pick a side. I wasn't looking for that even if they chose to take my side.

Similar to Dr. Gary, the social worker told me that what she was hearing was not unusual. In fact, she said that what I described was quite common. As it pertains to couples, she said that it's usually after treatment when all the emotions come out. She said that that's when things that you may not have noticed in each other before, start to become obvious. The little things that didn't bother us before, bothered us now. While Maddy and I were in treatment, the focus was on getting both of us through it and getting us well. As a couple, Brad and I didn't allow ourselves to pay or give attention to anything outside of that. Nothing else mattered. We didn't care about the nonsense we seem to fight about now. In other words, we "had bigger fish to fry." Everything else was just background noise that we were able to ignore. The social worker explained that now that the treatment is done for both my son and me, the focus shifts to all those things we ignored or suppressed. During my son's and my treatment, Brad and I hardly ever fought. We had tense moments for sure every now and then, due to the stress of the situation, but we never had these blow-ups that we've been having.

When I think about it, it makes sense. For the three years and a half years that Maddox was in treatment and for the half a year I was in treatment, we had one common goal that brought us together - to get Maddy and me in good health. For most couples, marriages naturally grow and evolve with time, and the relationship deepens. For Brad and me, our marriage took a back seat during that time. We are different people compared to the people we were when we first met. We are certainly not the same people we were before cancer changed our lives. Individually we have grown, matured, and changed, especially because of our circumstances. Together as a couple, maybe we have not. Because of that, our relationship has suffered. We didn't have time to nurture our marriage because we were too focused on taking care of our son and me. That was our priority. That's what mattered the most to us and rightly so. We didn't have room for anything else, much less our relationship.

I guess we are now dealing with the consequences of neglecting our marriage for so long. I can hear Dr. Del Toro's words when we sat down with him over four years ago, when he made references to many marriages not making it after dealing with the emotional stress of taking care of child in treatment. Could you imagine how much more stress is added when not just one, but two members of a family are stricken with cancer, at practically the same time?! Well, we didn't have to imagine it. We lived it. Back then, I brushed Dr. Del Toro's words aside, not really giving it any thought because I felt very secure in my marriage. Now, after having gone through and survived my son's treatment, and then my own, I can see and understand how easily a marriage can fall apart. In fact, I am amazed that Brad and I have held strong despite our marital issues. I think that's because at the very core of it all, is our love. No matter how often we fight or what we fight about, underneath it all, is pure, honest love. I truly believe that is what has held us together.

As I write this, Brad and I have only been married for nine years so far. In our young marriage, we have experienced a whole lot, more than most couples experience in a lifetime. We have weathered some really tough storms and it is not surprising that it has taken a toll on our relationship. Somehow, we always find a way back to each other. At our best, we are awesome together, a great match. I know in my heart that he is an amazing husband and father. He is my best friend and best partner. Oh, it's very true that at times we may not like each other very much, but the love, the love is always there. Perhaps only other married couples can appreciate and make sense of that.

Brad and I never made it to that counselor, but the fact that we got to that point made us take a close and hard look at our relationship. I think having that big blow up really shook both of us. We sure were damn close, but thank God we never crossed that line of no return. The fact that our marriage could get so fragile was a big wake-up call. I know that it scared me. The incident, our big blow-up, as contentious as it was at the time, really put things into perspective. I do have to admit that letting my emotions out in full force was quite cathartic. Once we realized how vulnerable our marriage was, we allowed ourselves to truly listen to each other. That's not to say that we stopped fighting after that. As with many married couples, there are still issues that come up that we argue about, and we still bicker every once in a while, but the difference is, there has been more of an effort on my part to step away when I'm feeling particularly moody and irritable. I am not always successful at it, but believe me, the effort is there. I hope my husband knows that. I think it's a work in progress for both of us. Since then, we are giving each other and our marriage the attention it has been missing for so long. It took a while, but in time, we found our rhythm once again.

Chapter Seventy-Seven

When you go through what we went through, it changes you. You become a different person. I'd like to think that in many ways I became a better version of myself. I would say, a much needed change from the person that I was before being diagnosed with breast cancer. Believe me, I know there is still work to be done. I am far from perfect. Yes, the events of the past recent years have certainly traumatized me, but I am doing my best to deal with the "emotional fallout." It would be impossible for someone to experience what I went through and not have some baggage. Despite the issues I am still working very hard to overcome, one thing is certain, I am incredibly grateful for this life.

Chapter Seventy-Eight

The Finish Line

In May of 2012, I finished my treatment. I would continue on tamoxifen for several more years, but my chemo and radiation days were done!

On a glorious day in August of 2012, Maddox finished his treatment!

There we were, Mother and Son, crossing the finish line.

I didn't make a big fuss of it when I finished my treatment. Throughout the whole process, with the exception of my family and a handful of close friends, I was really private about the whole thing. I honestly didn't want all the attention when I was done. All I wanted was just to quietly put it behind me. As grateful and happy as I was to be done with treatment, it meant more to me to celebrate the milestone privately with just my family. That was more than enough for me. I did not feel the need to make an announcement.

When Maddy finished his treatment, that was a different story. We wanted to shout it from the rooftops! That was an announcement that everyone deserved to hear because so many people took that journey with us. It was important to acknowledge and celebrate that amazing event with all the people that helped us get through it.

On August 28, 2012, with immeasurable love, gratitude, and joy in our hearts, we sent this message to all of our family and friends.

Hi Everybody,

We wanted to celebrate this very special occasion with all of you. After over 3 years and 2 months of treatment, Maddy got his last chemo at the clinic on Thursday, August 23rd, and got his last dose of chemo at home yesterday, Monday, August 27, 2012! We wanted to take this moment to thank all of you for the amazing support and love you have shown our family over these years.

We are beyond proud of our son. For everything he has been through, you would never know it. Maddox is kind and caring, with the most amazing sense of humor, and a laugh that puts a smile on your face every time. He has shown incredible courage and strength.

During Maddy's treatment, even after we settled into a "routine" of clinic visits, hospitalizations, and giving Maddy chemo at home every day, we never allowed ourselves to think back to those early days when he was diagnosed. Many of the memories were too painful and feelings of fear, heartache, and helplessness were just too much. We learned to live day to day, smiling through the tough times, focusing on the good and always, always looking forward, putting one foot in front of the other, determined to get to this day.

On the day of Maddy's last clinic chemo, sitting with the nurse with Maddy on my lap, ready to get his last dose of vincristine, Maddy must have referred to his IV as his "necklace." The nurse laughed and asked me how it came about that we called his IV, a necklace as she'd never heard it been called that before. Maddy was just a baby when he was diagnosed so Brad and I made up names so that Maddox wouldn't be scared. When he got his blood pressure, we called it "arm hugs," we referred to the clinic as, "The Kitchen" because there was a toddler kitchenette set that he loved to play with when he went in for his chemo, and so somehow, his IV came to be called a "necklace." I began to cry as I shared this with the nurse, and she and I told Maddy that today, Mommy has happy tears. In that instant, the significance of that moment came over me and as I watched the nurse administer Maddy's last chemo push, I was taken back to those early days and for the first time in a very long time, I allowed myself to remember.

It was in June of 2009 when Maddox was diagnosed with Acute Lymphoblastic Leukemia. Unprepared for what we were about to hear, Brad and I were in the hospital with Maddox when the Doctor comes in, sits across from us and says, "Maddox has leukemia." There was silence. In those few seconds, we probably stopped breathing. Then we fell apart. The only sound we heard was our uncontrollable crying as we held our son as tightly as we could. We cried for many days after that as we watched our son, only two and a half years old, subjected to exams, needles, x-rays, and tests. We felt helpless to stop it. As his parents, all we wanted was to just make it go away. Maddy was soon placed in protective isolation and would begin chemo immediately. As our family and friends came out in full force to support us, we managed to get it together. We learned a whole new language of CBC's and neutrophil counts and chemo medications. Once he completed his hospital treatment, we were able to bring him home. That was a great day. Those first few months of keeping Maddy in isolation at home and giving him chemo were not easy to say the least. He got chemo by mouth around the same time every day. There was also protocol we had to follow and precautions we had to take. While he was being treated, Maddy couldn't swim in the ocean or public pool, he was advised not to play in the sandbox or grass, he couldn't play contact sports, we had to plan play dates with caution, and he practically bathed in Purell whenever we went out. Through it all, Maddy never complained. Eventually, it just became part of what he knew, part of how we as a family adapted. It was Maddy's courage, that gave us strength.

As heartbreaking as some of the memories are of those first few weeks, believe it or not, there were also moments of humor. I remember one night when Maddy was on a heavy dose of steroids which made him ravenous...it must have been 3AM, lying next to him in the hospital bed, in the dark, when all I heard was him munching on an entire pack of sliced cheese! The steroids also made Maddy quite cranky. One day, Maddy was furiously demanding breakfast sausage. Well, it was dinner time and the cafeteria had no breakfast sausage so Grandma Shepard whipped up maybe two packs of sausage and walked almost two miles to the hospital to get Maddy his sausage. Yeah, we can laugh about it now! On another day, Maddy became curious about his mediport which is placed just under the skin on his chest and he said,

"Mommy, what is this?" I said, "That is your port so the doctors can give you your medicine." He replied, "Did I eat it?" I explained that the doctors put it there, but his logic was quite clever!

Because of this experience, we have come to appreciate the simple beauty of an ordinary day and we are so thankful for all that is good and simple.

As we take in the significance of this occasion, there are some special thanks we'd like to make.

We want to first and foremost Congratulate Maddox for his perseverance, courage, and strength! You are a brave kid! Well done, Maddox!

We want to thank our amazing daughter, Danika. It is the siblings that are often referred to as the unsung heroes in this fight. When she is old enough to understand, we will explain to her how much she sacrificed and didn't even realize it, to help take care of her big brother. Because Maddy had to be isolated at home for several months after being in the hospital, in order to protect him, Danika didn't go out either. Danika was Maddy's only play date and friend during those months of isolation. She was there for him. Because of the necessity of our circumstances, Maddy got most of our attention and we know that must have impacted her. She was just one and a half years old and didn't know what was going on. All she knew was that Mommy and Daddy were in and out of the apartment for weeks, each taking turns at home so that the other could be with Maddox at the hospital. Despite it all, Danika has shown Maddox so much love and compassion and we are so proud of her.

A huge thanks goes to Dr. Gustavo Del Toro, Maddox's oncologist at Mount Sinai. From the beginning, you never sugar coated anything for us. You prepared us for this fight and in the process, earned our utmost respect and trust. Most importantly, you earned Maddox's trust. In fact, whenever we needed Maddy to comply with taking his chemo or follow protocol, all we had to say was,

"Well, Dr. Del Toro says you have to do it" and he totally would do it - we thank you for that :) We all felt safe that Maddox was in your caring and capable hands.

Thank you to Dr. Wistinghausen, Megan, Rosie, Chrissy, Amy, Tanisha, Raj, Theresa, Lori, Vanessa, Mary Luz, Jeannette, Betty, Sara, Julia, and all the doctors, nurses, and staff at the Division of Pediatric Hematology and Oncology at Mount Sinai and at the pediatric hospital for taking such great care of Maddox, and for all the kindness you have shown our family while Maddy was being treated there.

Thank you to Dr. Gary Mason, Dr. Peter Steinherz, and the Peds team at Memorial Sloan Kettering Cancer Center for making Maddox's transition to MSKCC a smooth one, and especially for getting Maddox across the finish line!

Thank you to Linda, Mimi, Sheryl, and the entire Merricat's Castle School family. We are beyond grateful to all of you. Even with the precautions and limitations we had to take, it was a gift to have Maddy go to school and a gift to have some level of normalcy under our extraordinary circumstances. When Maddox was given the green light to go to school, you made sure to put certain protocols in place to keep him safe and because of that, the entire Merricat's community of parents and teachers came together to look after Maddy's well being so that he could enjoy school. We love you!

Thank you to Maddy's Kindergarten teachers, Ms. Ramona, Ms. Nicolo, Ms. Diaz, and Mr. Mike. You were so attentive with all of Maddy's precautions in school and always kept us informed whenever it was necessary so that we could keep Maddy safe. The kid loved Kindergarten - field trips galore! We are so thankful Maddox was able to participate in all of those events, knowing you all were looking after him.

Thank you to Barbara Zobian and Candlelighters for letting us know we were not alone in this fight. Together, through Candlelighters and with the amazing generosity of all of our family *and friends and the MetLife team, we have raised almost $50,000 over the past two years for The St. Baldrick's Foundation to support critical childhood cancer research and cure!*

Thank you to the Lodwig Family. You guys went above and beyond to support our family. You are awesome! You are our family.

The next two people that we want to thank are probably two of the most generous, selfless, kind-hearted, and loving people we know. With everything we feel in our hearts, we thank Dave and Cathie Shepard, our Mom and Dad. From day one, you never left our side. You came at a moment's notice whenever we needed you and even when we didn't. :) Your determination to get us through this was unwavering and so was your love and commitment to our family. We love you so much!

To all of our family, friends, and co-workers, with all of our hearts, we thank each and every one of you. As Brad and I reflect back on the past three years, we are overwhelmed with emotion. From the food and the toys that showed up at our home, to the incredibly generous donations made to the St. Baldrick's Foundation, the outpouring of support was truly moving. My mother-in-law has said to me that in tough times, God shows himself in others through acts of kindness. We knew we were not alone in this fight. You all lifted us up and we were strengthened every day by your love.

We have included an album which captures some of the moments of this journey. As we remember those moments and do our best to put them behind us, we do so with appreciation, because by allowing ourselves to take it all in, we allow ourselves to truly appreciate how far we've come. Maddy continues to be in remission and is doing well. Please keep him in your prayers for continued good health.

Today is the first day that Maddy is chemo free! It is the first ordinary day we've had in a very long time. Ordinary is good. Ordinary feels amazing!

We celebrate this achievement with all of you!

Love,
Brad, Geri, Maddox and Danika

After I sent that e-mail announcing Maddox's last day of chemo and treatment, the numerous, countless responses we got were filled with so much love and jubilance. Everyone shared in our joy and it felt wonderful.

Here are some of the many beautiful messages that we received.

Congratulations MADDY! I was so choked up reading your email last night and I struggled to write a response to your gorgeous, eloquent tribute to your family. The photographs were so incredibly touching, any distant observer would be able to see the strength and love and bravery in the eyes of two parents, a little sister and an innocent little child. What a gift it has been for everyone you thanked in your email to have been associated with The Shepard Family!

How amazing it is. I am so happy that this journey has been triumphant for Maddox. You have amazing children. I am impressed by your stories. Your family is inspiring.

Thank you so much for sharing a very personal and what must have been emotional part of your life with us. I must say, that your family is one of the main reasons I enjoy what I do. Watching the dynamics of your family and support, knowing this journey was an unexpected ball thrown out of left field, in which you all were able to come together and reorganize your lives and not let it take over, but instead entwine it and make it almost seem normal, is such an accomplishment in itself. We are so happy to know that Maddy is doing well and has completed treatment.

'Ordinary' has never sounded so good.

So happy that you and your family have closed that chapter of life. Wishing you guys the best, and a happy, healthy future.

What an amazing blessing, Geri, mazel tov in the biggest way possible.

Hooray for Maddy and for all of you. Congratulations! I cannot imagine your emotions, but I can say that one true gift was that we all got to know you and your incredible family. You and Brad are an amazing couple, to have survived and somehow manage to thrive and always have a smile and warm greeting and hug for all you meet, no matter what you were facing and struggled with. We love your family dearly and feel honored and loved for you to have allowed us be a part of your family and your lives.

I'm so glad that Maddy is done with his treatment. It is truly amazing what strength he had through all of this at such a young age. And also how Danika was so supportive and his "best friend" during this time. Maddy is truly a special kid.

I'm so truly happy for Maddox and your family. You guys are a true inspiration of what love can do. With tears in my eyes I shared this letter with my team as it reminded me that all the work they do means something amazing. Hopefully I can be ½ as good a mother as you are.

You've thanked everyone else, but you and Brad are the ones I hold responsible for this wonderful outcome as well as for the way all of your lives will now continue. The love you two generate touches all who come into contact with it.

Your letter of celebration is amazing--so much thought, caring, love, dedication, endurance. God bless you for all your family has endured, survived and been able to grow together to emerge healthy and smiling.

Oh Geri, what a beautiful tribute to your amazing little boy. Congratulations, Maddy!! It is so incredible to sense the genuine smile behind your words as your sweet boy reaches this milestone. What a journey. And what an incredible family you have, Geri. I am absolutely moved to tears by the strength of your character and the love in your heart that helped carry your family through this.

God Bless you guys and God Bless Maddox, what a hero! You go Maddox! You are an inspiration! Way to kick cancer's ass! Now go out there and change the world kid! You earned it and you deserve it! You and Brad are an inspiration too, he is strong because you guys are strong & courageous, now you see where he gets it!

These are some of the photos that we included in our e-mail.

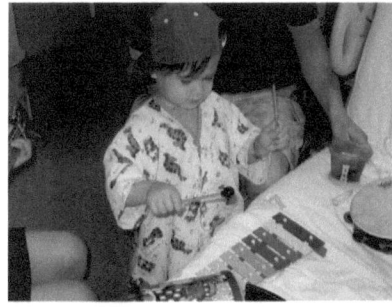
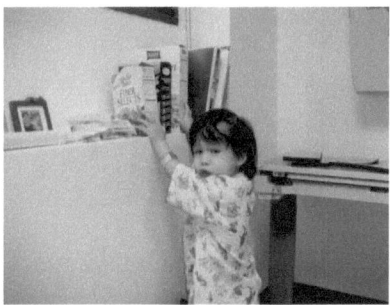

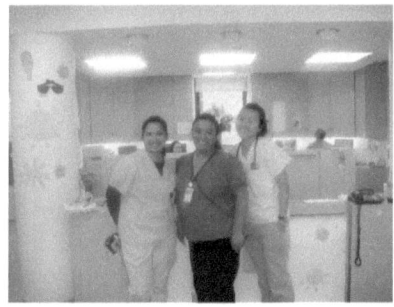
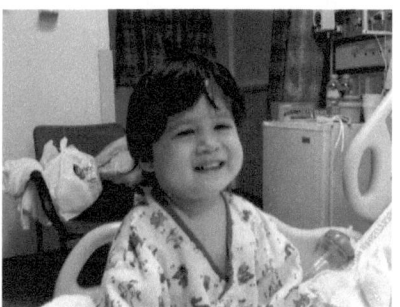

The Wonderful Mount Sinai Nurses.   Discharge Day!

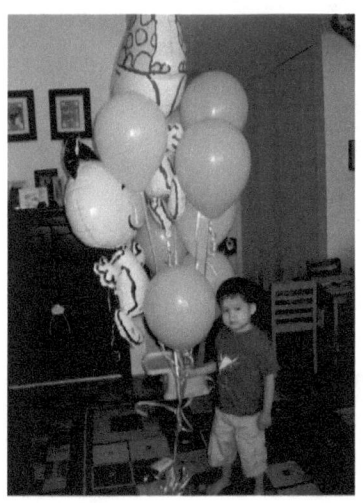
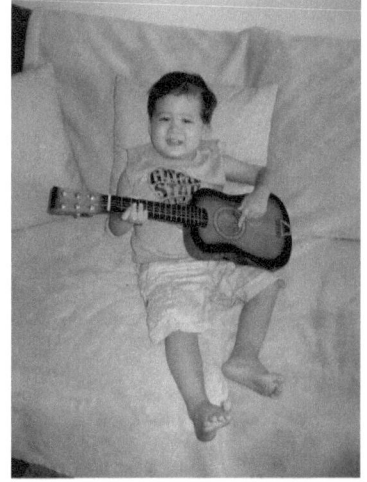

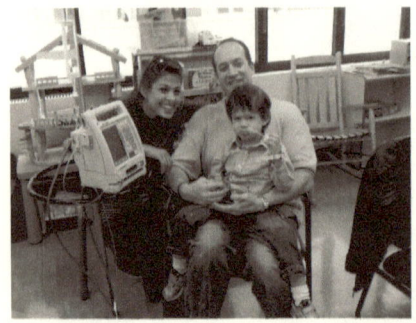
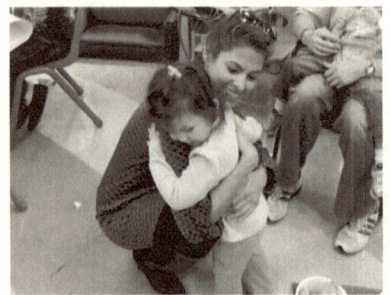

Maddox and Danika meet movie star, Eva Mendes.

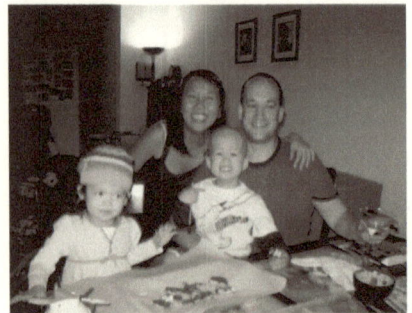
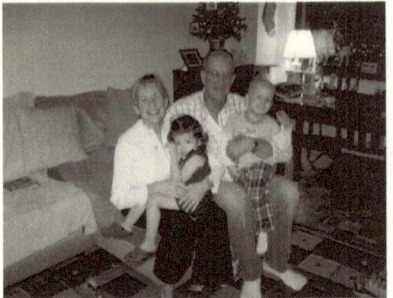

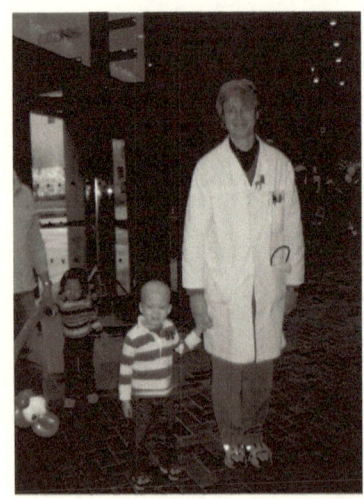
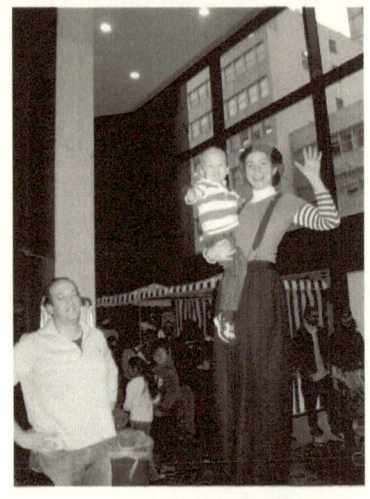

Dr. Del Toro, Our Fearless Leader.   Mount Sinai Holiday Party.

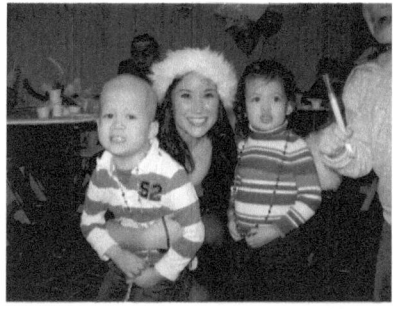 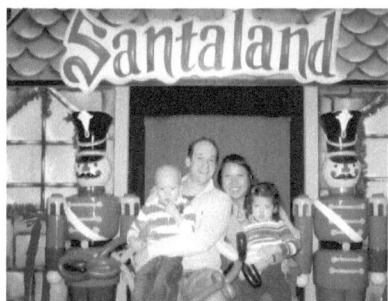

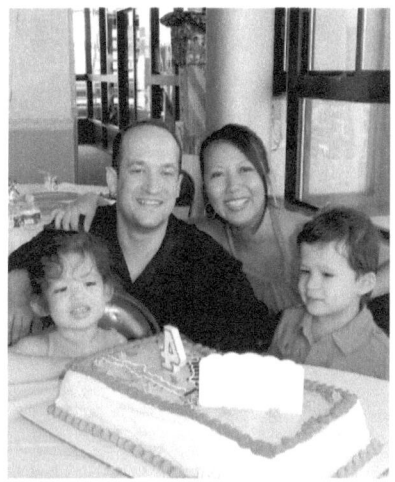 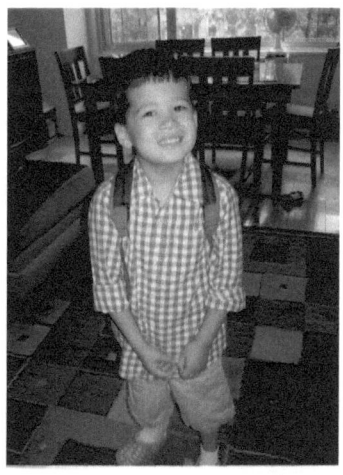

First Day of Kindergarten.

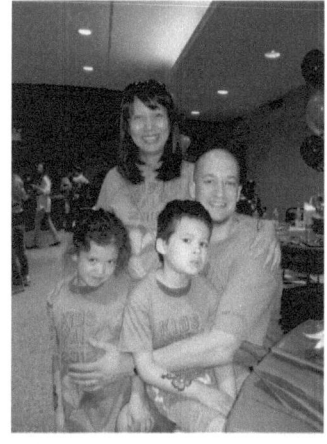 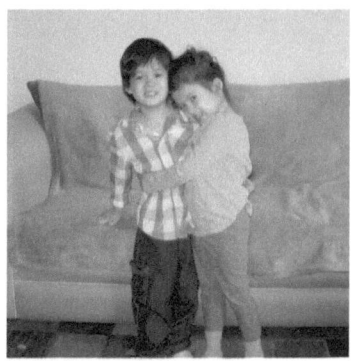

Bye Bye Yuckies!   Best Friends.

Geri Payawal Shepard

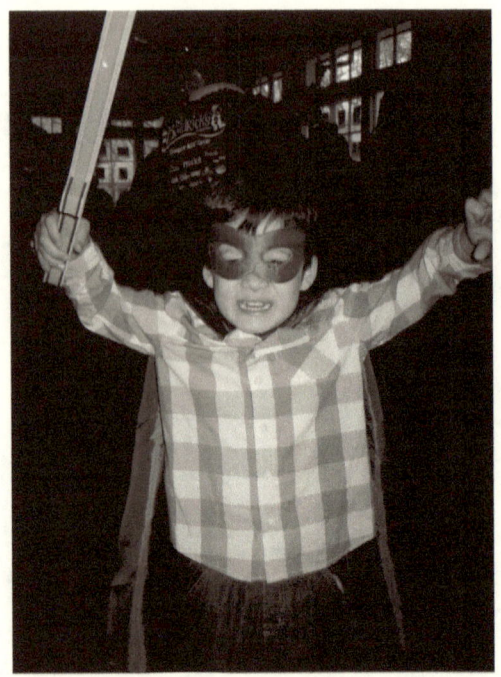

Our Little Hero.

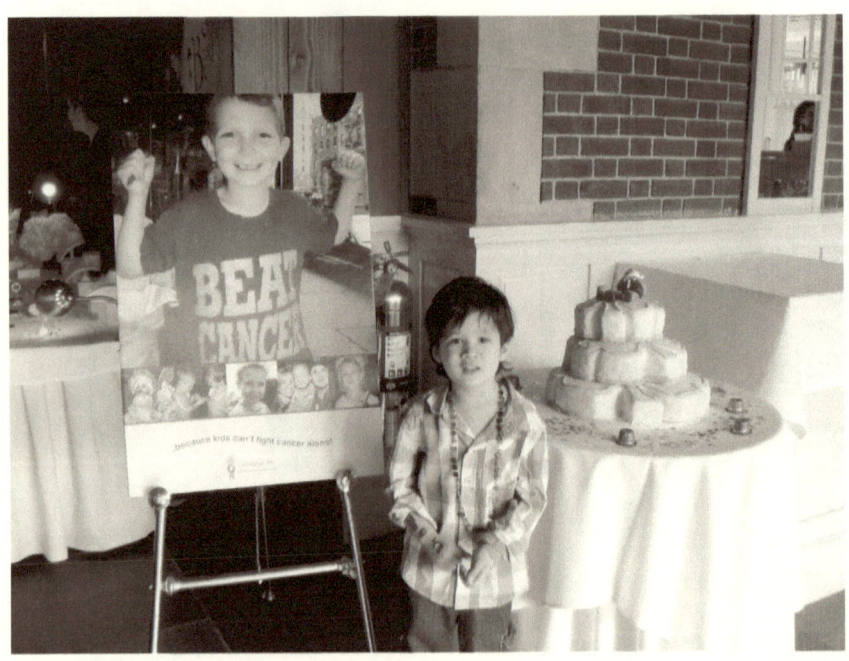

Chapter Seventy-Nine

After three and a half long years, the first day that I didn't have to prepare Maddy's chemo was the day a tremendous weight was finally lifted off of my shoulders. I was free. I remember at one point looking at the clock. It would have been the time to get Maddy' chemo prepared, but that day, that amazing day, I didn't have to do a damn thing. The significance of that moment was not lost on me as I said a very heartfelt silent prayer of thanks. That night, in honor of Maddy finishing his chemo treatment, we took the family out for a special pizza dinner. I tell ya, pizza never tasted as delicious as it did that night.

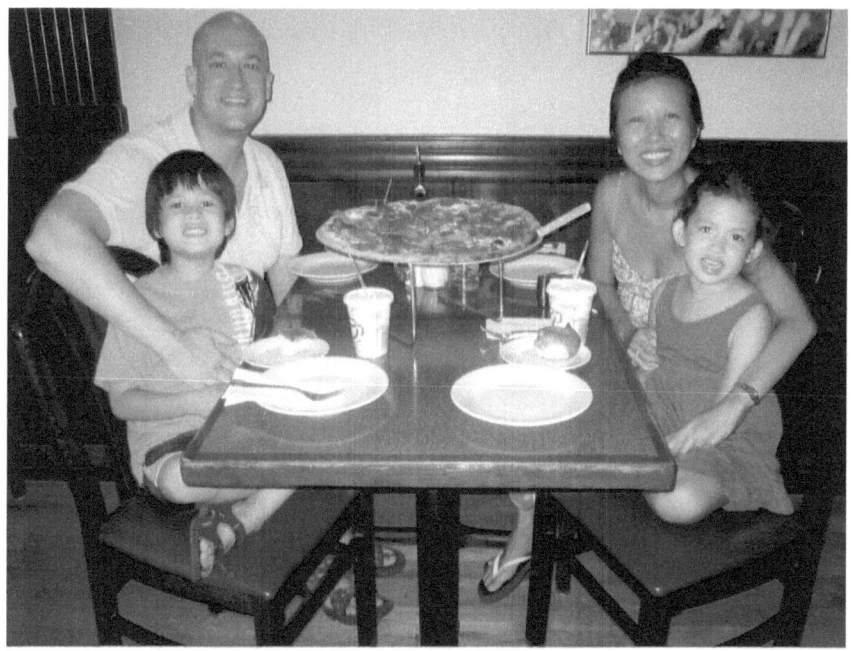

Pizza Celebration Party!

Chapter Eighty

September 5, 2012

On this wonderful day, Maddy had surgery to remove his mediport.

It was a fairly routine and quick operation, but I always had a level of anxiety whenever Maddy had to be sedated for a procedure. We would be allowed in the room only up until Maddy was put under. I knew that I only had a moment to give Maddy a hug and a kiss, and tell him that I loved him before they administered that white milky substance. It was always quite amusing to watch Maddy get the anesthesia. Maddy would get this loopy, dopey smile on his face right before he fell asleep. It literally took only a matter of seconds before Maddy was completely out.

Each and every time that Maddy had to get a procedure, I would sit quietly in the waiting room praying that everything would go smoothly. This time was no different. Dr. Gary was there to oversee the removal of the port. After about twenty minutes, he came out to tell us that all went well. Thank you Lord! Now all we had to do was wait. Dr. Gary sat with us the whole time waiting for Maddy to come out of the anesthesia. I knew he wanted to be there to share in this incredibly momentous occasion. While finishing chemo marked the completion of Maddy's treatment, getting his port removed made it even more official.

I remember Brad and I sitting outside the procedure room, waiting for Maddy to wake up. We were very quiet. I knew that we were both thinking about this long journey and what it took for us to get where we finally were. As I sat there, I relived many of the moments that I would have rather forgotten. I was a jumble of emotions struggling to keep it under control. It was as if all the events of the past three and half years, along with all the emotions that went with them flashed before my eyes. We have been through so much to get to this point. The port was where Maddy was accessed to administer the chemo and other drugs. Having his port finally removed symbolized the end of this journey. That's a *huge* deal. We made it here. In a moment of clarity, as I waited for my brave son to emerge from the room, I realized that we really survived it. Three and a half long years. Wow.

After about 45 minutes, the door opened and a very groggy and slightly wobbly Maddy walked out of the recovery room. He was a such beautiful sight. Instantly, Brad and I were on our feet rushing to our son. With both of us crying, overwhelmed by our emotions, we held onto Maddy and each other for a very long time. These were very, very happy tears. As I'm writing this, I couldn't help but remember that day, years ago when we all held each other like that when Maddy was diagnosed, only then the mood was quite different, quite somber. Now fast forward three and a half years later, there we were, holding each other once again, this time in pure JOY. Overcome with gratitude and sweet relief, I said, "You did it, Maddy! You did it." I could feel the nurses and Dr. Gary watching us and they too were teary-eyed as they watched our family embrace. All of those long years of heartache, challenges, and victories culminated in this profound moment. We were really done.

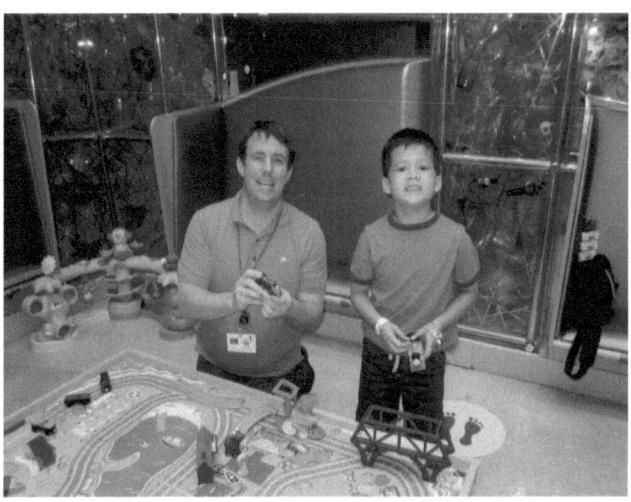

Maddy with Dr. Gary after his port is removed!

Chapter Eighty-One

After Maddox and I finished our treatments, it was time to celebrate!

In October of 2012, with Grandma Shepard babysitting the kids, Brad and I took a much needed couple's vacation to Puerto Rico, staying at the posh St. Regis Resort. Amazing. We were actually on *vacation*. For several years, it was a concept that had become foreign to us, and now there we were, appreciating and soaking in every delicious moment. Brad and I had spent so many years focused on taking care of our son, then taking care of me, now it was time to focus on each other.

Our marriage took a back seat for many years while we dealt with the unimaginable. This trip allowed us to celebrate the love that got us through it. There's no question that I have been through a lot, but so has Brad. To stand by your family as your son, and then your wife go through cancer treatment took an enormous amount of strength. A lesser man would have checked out, but not Brad. He loved us through everything.

They say it is easy to love someone when things are going well. It is during the tough times that the strength of that love is truly revealed. I'd say that Brad and I have proven our love to be strong and steady. Our vows have certainly been tested in the recent past years and through it all, the challenges and our victories, Brad and I have honored the sacred promises of love and commitment we made to each other on our wedding day.

Brad and I were so ready for this vacation. While Brad enjoyed the pool, I often took some time for myself to sit on the beach and think about the past recent years. I find myself doing that more often than I'd like. Many of the memories bring me to tears and the heartache and pain would feel like a fresh wound. But it was time to heal and leave those memories far, far behind in order to make room for new and happy ones. Being in this paradise was a great start.

Brad and I spent five blissful days luxuriating in our surroundings. Each day, admiring the beautiful view of serene waters and clear skies, I would take several deep, long breaths in appreciation of all things good. I think of my affectionate and loyal husband, my brave and kind-hearted Maddy-moo, and my smart and sassy Danzi-roo. They are what matter most to me in this world. I close my eyes and just breathe, savoring every delicious moment as if I was breathing new life into my body. I felt healthy and I felt strong. As I listened to the soft waves of the ocean and welcomed the warmth of the sun on my face, and fresh sea breeze on my body, all I could do was be grateful, simply grateful that we were there. This vacation gave Brad and I the opportunity to reconnect and more especially, to count our blessings.

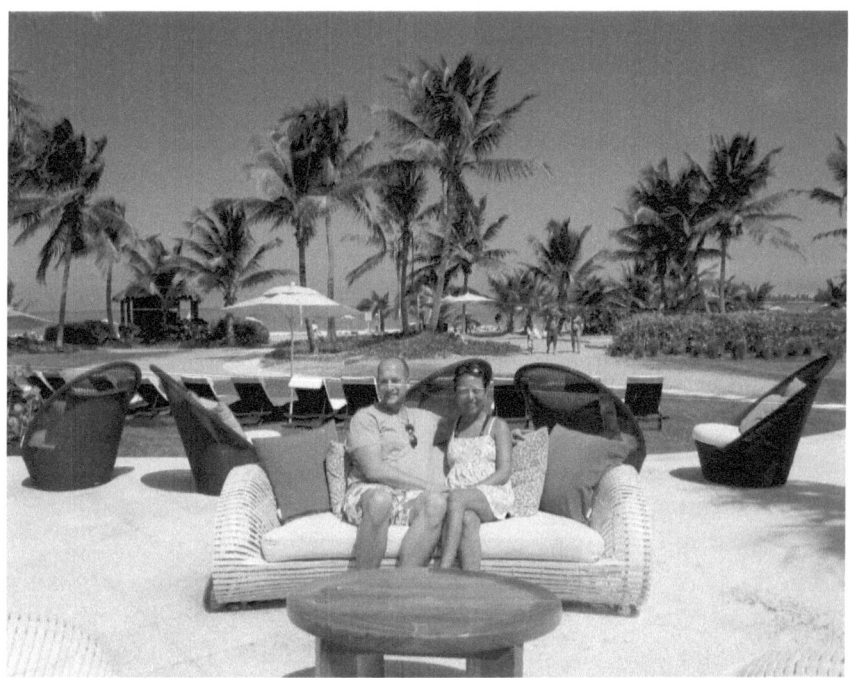

Paradise in Puerto Rico.

Chapter Eighty-Two

A couple of short weeks after that wonderful vacation, feeling renewed and rejuvenated, I walked in the Making Strides Against Breast Cancer Walk. While many of my family and friends generously donated to my fundraising efforts, I didn't form a team or invite anyone to walk with me. I wanted to do it on my own. I didn't want to make a big deal about it. It's hard to explain why. All I can say is that it was something I was doing for myself and I wanted to do it privately - among of course thousands of people. I liked the anonymity of walking among strangers bonded together for a common cause.

That morning, I was given a sash that read, "Survivor." Powerful word. When the walk began, I was surrounded by a sea of pink. The crowd was massive, as well as inspirational, with every person there in support of putting an end to breast cancer. Damn, right! My intention was to walk quietly by myself. Along the way, while I didn't plan on meeting anyone, I happened to befriend one woman in particular. I don't remember her name, but that day we somehow gravitated towards each other, and in the process, shared our stories as we walked several miles together. We also bonded over the character, Kristina, in the show, *Parenthood*. The show told the story of Kristina's breast cancer journey. The actress, Monica Potter, played the part with such honesty and integrity. I remember watching the show thinking, "Oh my gosh, that's exactly what I went through" and "I know exactly what she's feeling." It felt so close to home that it was as if this character, Kristina, was telling my own story. It was cathartic to watch it, cry with it, relate to it - just as it was cathartic to confide in this woman that I had just met. We had both been through a lot and like me, she chose to do the walk alone, without the fanfare of any family or friends walking beside us. She understood. I know the word "private" is a strange way to describe an event that is anything but private, but that's what it was for us.

I remember walking the route hearing the roar of hundreds of people on the sidelines applauding and cheering for us. Many of them would read my sash and in show of support, would shout, "SURVIVOR!" The first time I heard it yelled out to me, I was jolted. It was like a moment of truth hitting me with such a force that it brought me to tears. Wow, they were talking about *me*. I could see the look of admiration in so many of their nameless faces. It was incredibly moving. It made me remember everything I went through and suffered during my treatment. I was knocked down more times than I'd care to remember, but somehow, I always, always got back up. I AM a Survivor. I was overcome with emotion, and as the tears wet my cheeks, I welcomed the praise and acknowledgment. I earned it. I wore that sash with pride. There was so much love and support in the air. It felt good and I was so glad to have been a part of this walk.

After I crossed the finish line, I found Brad, Maddox, and Danika waiting for me with big smiles on their faces. It was for them that I fought so hard to get through it. Their love gave me strength. As my husband and children ran up to me, my arms were wide open to welcome their hugs and kisses. My heart was full. This walk was an incredibly moving experience and a very meaningful way for me to close this chapter in my story.

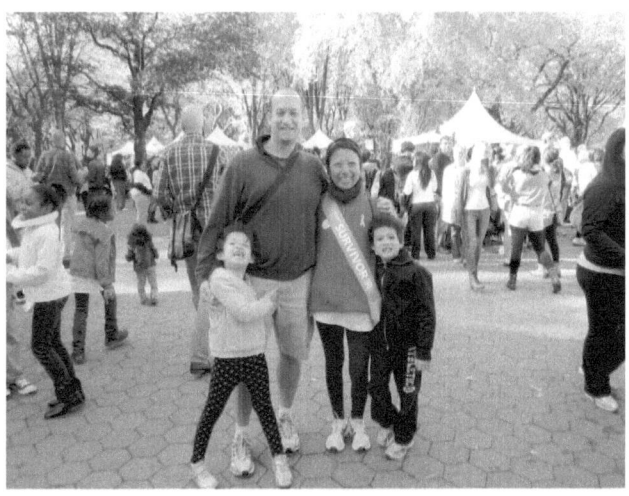

Making Strides Against Breast Cancer Walk 2012.

Chapter Eighty-Three

I was so ready to make some new and joyful memories. We all were. There was no better way to do that than to go on another vacation!

In May of 2011, I contacted the Make-A-Wish foundation in the hopes of getting a wish granted for Maddox. I had recently heard about another family who had just been granted a wish and I thought it would be a wonderful experience for Maddox to have as well. On my initial call, a very kind woman went through a series of questions about Maddox's medical history. The woman asked what Maddy's diagnosis was and as I began to reply, I felt all of this emotion resurface. All of a sudden, I found my eyes welling up and my voice cracking as I answered, "Acute Lymphoblastic Leukemia." I was taken aback by own emotions. By this time, I thought I had told our story enough times or that I had built a strong enough wall that I could just simply answer the questions, but there was nothing simple about it. My son had leukemia. I guess for me, that topic will never not be emotional. I had to take a moment to compose myself and steady my voice so that I could continue the call. The woman was very kind and patient as I apologized in between tears. I'm sure I'm not the only parent who has cried on the phone with her when discussing their child's illness. It must be quite daunting to hear all of those emotional stories, but at the same time, it must be incredibly rewarding to know that you are a part of bringing joy to many of the families. Once we were done, she explained that MAW would contact Mount Sinai to get more information to complete our application. Julia, the social worker at Mount Sinai, assisted with submitting all the requested medical documents, as well as the signed consent form from Dr. Del Toro to MAW.

It wasn't long after our application was fully submitted that we met with a couple of Make-A-Wish representatives to discuss Maddox's wish. The representatives, Christina and Matt came to our home to meet Maddox and our family. When they called to schedule the meeting, they asked about what kinds of toys Maddy liked and of course, we told them that he absolutely loves anything related to Thomas the Train. When they arrived at our door, they handed Maddox a present and sure enough it was a Thomas toy. It was so thoughtful for them to have done that. At the meeting, Christina and Matt told us about all the different kinds of wishes that could be granted, like meeting a celebrity or having a party. While there were many great wishes, the one wish we all agreed would be perfect for our whole family, was a trip to Walt Disney World. They told us that it was one of the most popular requests and rightfully so. That wish would be a wonderful gift not just for Maddox, but for Danika as well. For all that she has sacrificed to take care of her big brother, Danika was just as deserving of a special experience. After everything we've been through, it was a wonderful wish that our whole family could appreciate and enjoy.

Once we decided on the trip, the wish had to go through an approval process. In the meantime, pending approval, they wanted to get an idea on when we would like to go on the trip. As much as we would have loved to have gone right away, we told them that we would prefer to go once Maddox finished his treatment. We wanted Maddox to be able to fully enjoy this vacation without having to be limited by the many restrictions he had to follow. I also did not want the burden of bringing all of his chemo and all the gear that went with it, on the trip. That would have been a real drag. If we went during his treatment, we would have also had to consider what would happen, God forbid, if Maddy got sick on the trip. With Maddy on chemo, his immune system would still be compromised. We'd spend the whole time worrying about whether or not Maddy was going to catch any germs. Could you imagine how many times I would have to Purell Maddy's hands in one of the largest and most public amusement parks known to man?! No thank you! If Maddy got a fever, we would have to take him to a hospital that we weren't familiar with, and then we'd have to go through the whole process of going over Maddox's medical history and medications. The thought of that was just too daunting. I would not risk putting Maddox and our family through that.

A long time ago, a very nice mom told me about MAW sending her family to either Disney World or Disney Land. I can't remember which one. They decided to take the trip while their daughter was still in treatment. For their own personal reasons, it was a decision that worked best for them. I remembered the mom telling me that in the middle of the trip they had to go back home because their daughter got sick. Her daughter and their family had a wonderful time while they were there, but I'm sure having to cut their trip short was certainly no fun. I never forgot that story, so when it came to picking potential dates for our trip, I knew without a shadow of a doubt, and with complete certainty, that it had to be after Maddy's treatment was finished. Absolutely.

When we discussed our desired travel dates with Christina and Matt, Maddox still had about a year and a half of treatment left. While it seemed like long time to wait, Brad and I were more than confident that it was the right decision. With Maddy's treatment done and behind us - that was the only way we could all truly enjoy this amazing wish. Knowing that a spectacular vacation was waiting for us at the end of this long journey somehow made each day until then just a little bit easier. This trip would be something for us to look forward to, something that would keep our focus and determination straight ahead. Eyes on the prize, baby. When I say prize, I mean Maddy finishing his treatment. That was the ultimate prize. Going to Disney would be the icing on the cake.

Chapter Eighty-Four

Disney World

In July of 2011, we got the official word from Christina, the wish coordinator, that Maddox's wish was granted. AWESOME!!! We eagerly set our travel dates for the following year. It seemed like a long way off, but for us, this trip would be our bright sun in the horizon.

On November 10, 2012, three months after Maddox completed his treatment, we were on our way to Disney World!!!

This vacation was beyond anything we could have dreamed up. It was everything and more.

We wanted to surprise the kids so we didn't mention anything about the trip. I packed all of our bags the night before and I hid them so they wouldn't suspect a thing. For several weeks before that, Brad and I immersed them in all things Mickey, Minnie, and Disney that was on the Disney channel. They had never been to Disney World before - much less any place else. For the three and a half years Maddy was in treatment, we did not go on any vacations or travel anywhere that required a plane trip. Up until then, the only amusement park they've ever been to was Victorian Gardens in Central Park. It was a really nice, but small park for toddlers and young children, with just a handful of rides. The kids really loved going there. Now, they were about to go to Disney, the grand daddy of all amusement parks! Boy, they were in for such a treat! Brad and I could hardly contain our own excitement.

The morning of our trip, Brad and I tiptoed into the kids' bedroom and woke them up yelling, "Surprise! We're going to Disney World!!!" To be honest, we didn't quite get the reaction we were expecting. We thought there would be immediate squeals of joy, but instead they just gave us looks of bewilderment. They knew something good was happening, but they didn't really quite get it yet. As I mentioned, we haven't traveled or been on a vacation in over three years. The kids were familiar with Disney because they watched Disney Junior, but they weren't quite sure what Disney World actually was. We didn't show them the Disney World travel video because we wanted the trip to be a surprise. Brad and I quickly explained to them that we were going to a place where they would get to meet Mickey, Minnie, and Goofy, and go on lots of rides, and where we would go on lots of amazing adventures. I told Danika she would get to meet all the princesses and even get to go inside Cinderella's castle. Well, it didn't take very long for these kids to whip off their pajamas in pure excitement. Their faces were beaming with huge smiles of delight. Now we're talkin'!

With the kids dressed and raring to go, we got picked up in style. Compliments of MAW, a long stretch limo pulled up in front of our building to whisk us off to the airport. Yup - a limo! Maddox and Danika couldn't believe that this fancy car was just for us. I must admit, it made me feel pretty special too. Our chauffeur took our bags and opened the door for us like we were celebrities! The kids were all giggles and they got such a big kick out of how big the limo was inside. I literally sat several feet away from them on the other side of the limo to take their pictures. They thought it was the neatest thing ever, and our wish was only just beginning. We would soon find out just how much the MAW Foundation did to make Maddox's wish as wondrous and magnificent as it could be - for all of us.

On the ride to the airport and on the plane, Maddox kept singing, "We're going to Disney World! We're gonna see Mickey and Minnie and Goofy. We're going to Disney World!" It was quite amusing. When we arrived in Orlando, we were greeted by a gentleman carrying a sign with Maddox's name on it. He escorted us to our rental car, which again was compliments of MAW, and gave us directions to Give Kids the World Village, a "storybook resort" that would be our accommodations for the week. This was all part of our wish package. Give Kids the World is an amazing organization that provides resort accommodations and all meals at no cost to the MAW families. Their mission is to fulfill the wishes of these children and provide them and their families with a joy-filled vacation. As soon as we pulled up to the Village, I knew we were in for something truly special. We were all excited to explore the resort, but our first stop was to check-in at the front office. There I received our welcome packet. I scheduled the orientation for later that afternoon. Inside the office, we got a glimpse of what was outside the doors and we all got very excited. We could barely keep the kids from racing outside, so after we finished checking in, and before we got settled into our room, we decided to do a quick walk-through of the Village area just outside the office.

When we opened those doors, it was like stepping into an enchanted land. Everything was so colorful and vibrant, almost as if we walked right into a fairy tale. This was a place where your imagination could really soar. There was a child sized train ride, buildings that looked like gingerbread houses, Elmer the talking and snoring tree, a merry-go-round, a gorgeous pool, and even an all day ice cream parlor that served ice cream for breakfast! That was just one part of the Village. It went on and on. We walked around in pure joy and awe. Give Kids the World Village was more than a resort, it was its own amusement park! There was so much to take in and we hadn't even unpacked our bags yet. As much as we wanted to see everything, it was time to get settled in our room.

The kids and I got into this golf cart like car with our Village representative, who escorted us to our accommodations. I think Brad followed behind in our rental car. As we drove, I noticed all of these quaint little homes. I thought we would be staying in a hotel room, but as we approached our destination, I realized we actually would have our very own cottage! In fact, all of the families were given these homes. When you looked around the street, each cottage was a different color, with its own porch in front. It was like our own whimsical neighborhood. There was a sign in front of our house with our name, "Shepard" on it. So delightful! When we first walked into the cottage, there were presents on the kitchen table waiting for the kids. They of course, immediately and excitedly tore them open. The representative told us that the gift fairy came every day to deliver presents so that every day, when we arrived home, there would be new presents on the table waiting for both Maddox and Danika. Amazing! The kids were beaming. My heart was filled with so much joy. Inside the cottage were two bedrooms, two bathrooms, our very own fully equipped kitchen, and a living room. It would be our home for the week and it was awesome!

In addition to the gift fairy, the rep told us that the Village hosted a theme party every night, complete with games and a delicious assortment of sweet treats. She went on to say that there would be horse rides at the corral, that every day there would be special visits from our favorite Disney characters, including Mickey Mouse himself, for photos and autographs, and then, per request, Mayor Clayton of the Village - which by the way, was a life-size bunny - would even tuck the kids in at bedtime! These were just some of the many wonderful activities and events offered at the Give Kids the World Village. Fantastic!!!!

I thought I had heard it all, then I went to the orientation. Since they didn't require that we all be present for the orientation, it gave Brad and the kids the opportunity to explore the rest of the Village. At the orientation, I sat with a small group, each one of us representing our families, as the GKTW rep went through all of the material in our welcome packet. I should note that many, if not all of the staff and representatives at GKTW, are volunteers. It warmed my heart to know that so many of the people working in the Village, including our orientation rep were there out of the kindness of their hearts. Our speaker was a sweet-faced older gentleman and it was obvious to me that he took great pleasure in what he was doing. He was a part of this caring organization that brings joy to so many families and when he spoke to us, you could tell he shared in that joy. He was just as thrilled as us to get to the good stuff. As instructed, I took out all the items from the packet and for a moment, just stared at everything, half in disbelief, half in amazement. I knew our wish was a trip to Disney World, I just had no idea that it included so many incredible perks!

As the rep went through and explained each item, I was awestruck. In front of me were complimentary tickets to Magic Kingdom, to

Epcot, Hollywood Studios, Animal Kingdom, and SeaWorld. The rep particularly highlighted a special ID badge for one of the family members to wear to all the parks so that we didn't have to wait on any long lines for the rides and attractions. This badge would communicate to all the park employees that we were a Wish family. There was a GKTW pin for Maddox to wear so that the park staff would immediately know he was a Wish child. The rep went on to explain that all the park employees were well aware of the significance of the badge and the pin, and would immediately know to escort us straight to the front of any line. Wow. Once again, WOW! My excitement was building wanting to burst listening to this kind man explain that all of these wonderful benefits were for us. All of it was more than we could have ever dreamed of and we hadn't even gone through everything in the packet yet.

The perks continued. We were given passes for free parking every day we went to one of the parks. There was a coupon to get a free photo at SeaWorld and best of all, there was a complimentary Disney Photopass worth almost $200 that allowed us to have unlimited photos taken at all the Disney parks. No freakin' way! YES, way!!! We could capture as many memories as we wanted and we didn't have to pay for a single picture. Anyone who knows me knows how much I love a good photo! Let's continue. MAW also provided us with a generous stipend to spend on food and souvenirs. Then to top it all off, we were presented with a certificate that granted all four of us free admission to any participating theme and amusement park, good for one year after our Disney trip. AMAZING!!! This wish truly was the gift that just kept on giving. I think it was right around the time the rep was explaining the Disney Photopass, that I started to cry. As he went through each item, one great gift after another, I felt so much love. I was incredibly moved by the profound generosity and thoughtfulness that went into granting our family this grand and splendid wish. Sitting there, I thought about everything we have been through to get to this day, to this moment. I took it all in and just felt grateful, so grateful to be where we were. Yeah, we deserved this trip and it felt great.

As the orientation wrapped up, I looked around and noticed a woman sitting just a few seats next to me. Like me, she too was crying. I understood. She was probably just as blown away as I was at the tremendous generosity of our hosts. We each went through and survived our own hell and we were more than ready to welcome happiness back into our lives. As we prepared to leave, this woman got up, gathered her belongings, went straight to our rep, and hugged him. I was right behind her. Our families just received the most amazing gift and we both wanted to express how thankful we were for everything, and it was so much. We caught each others eyes, both of us with joyful tears, and without any words, we just smiled. It made me realize even more that every family there had a story to tell. I know this vacation meant the world to all of us. Make-A-Wish and Give Kids The World didn't just give us a trip, they gave us a truly special experience that we will never forget.

After the orientation, I met up with Brad and the kids. They had discovered a Candy Land themed playground and the kids couldn't get enough of it. This place was every child's fantasy! I told Brad about the orientation and he too was impressed by everything our trip included. That night, we attended our first Village party. It was a pool party with lots of food, games, and cotton candy! Brad and I sat on the pool chairs simply content watching our beautiful kids so carefree and happy. We needed this. I didn't realize how much so until we were sitting there taking it all in. Maddox and Danika were having the best time with huge, mega-watt smiles on their faces. As parents, there is no greater joy than that. Later that evening, Mayor Clayton of the Village and his wife, Ms. Merry, made an appearance thrilling all of the children who quickly ran up to greet and hug them. After all, it is only in this wondrous place that we got to have a life-size bunny as Mayor. We could have partied all night with them, but we had to rest up. We had a very big day the next day. Before we hit the sack, Maddy entertained us with another song and dance about Disney World. We went to bed that night grateful beyond measure. Mickey, here we come!

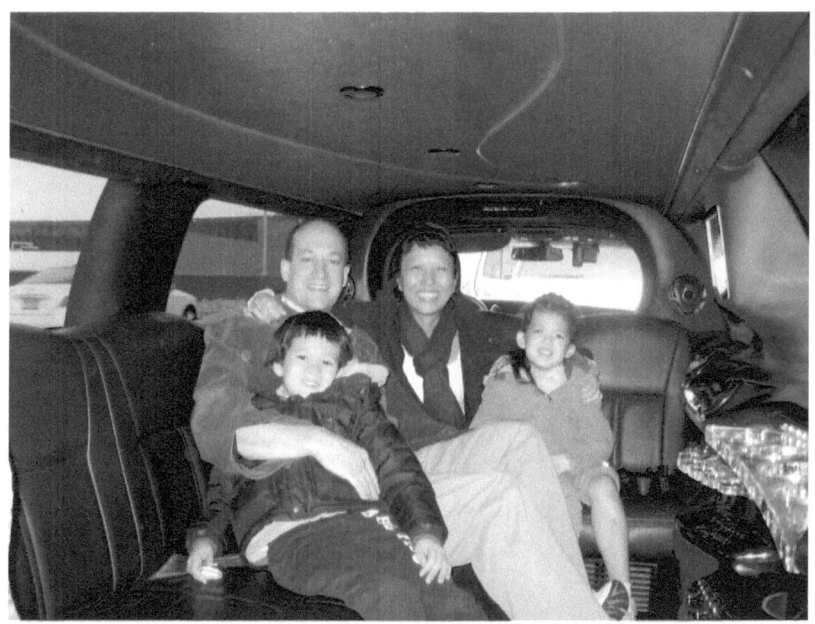

We're going to Disney World!

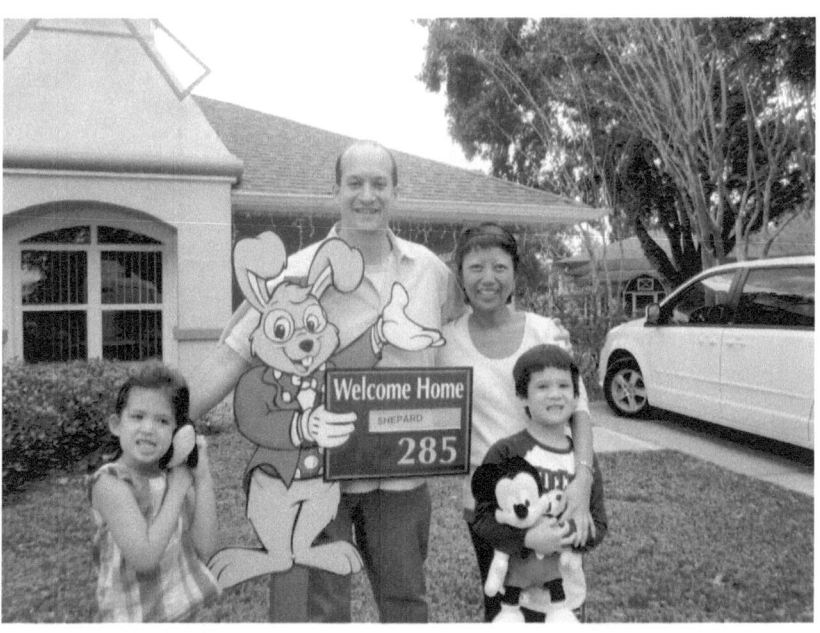

Our Fairy Tale Cottage at Give Kids the World Village.

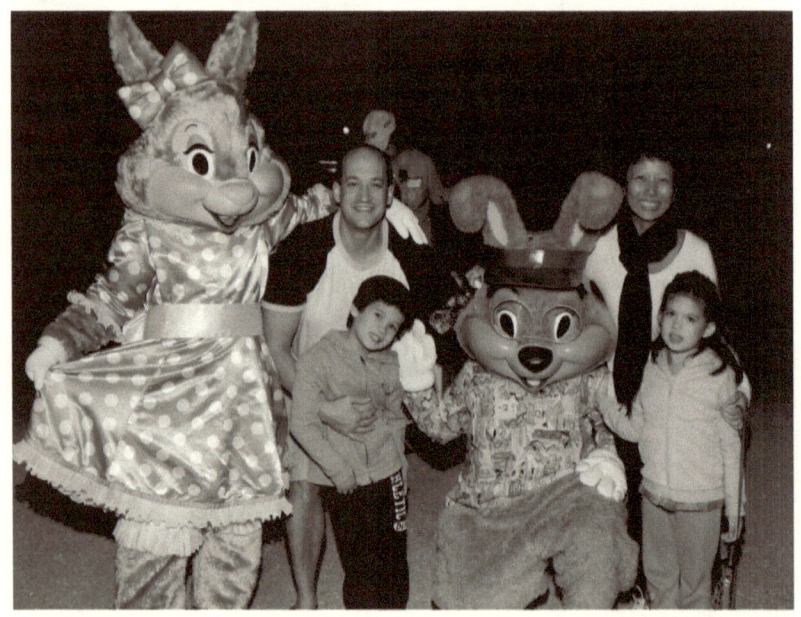

Village Pool Party with Mayor Clayton and his wife, Ms. Merry.

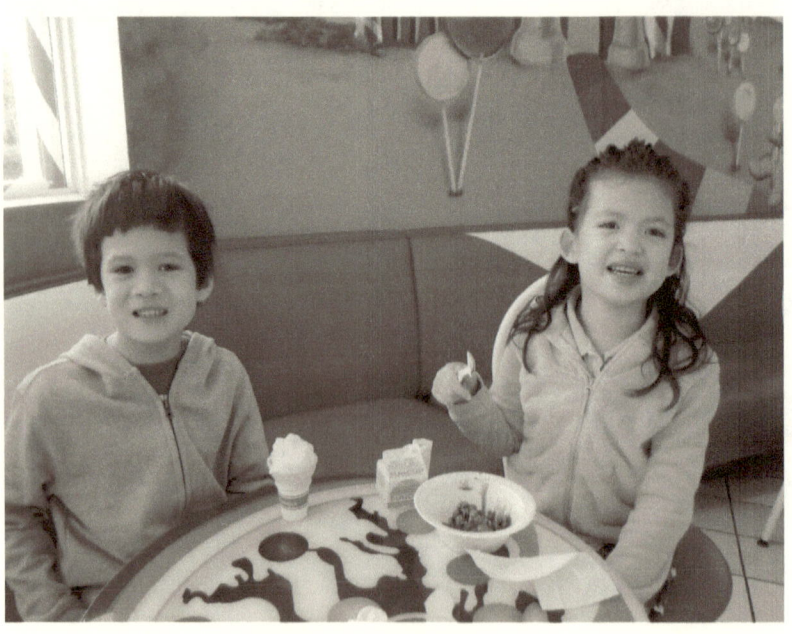

Ice Cream for Breakfast!

Chapter Eighty-Five

We woke up the next morning filled with eagerness and anticipation. In keeping with the Village tradition, Maddox and Danika had ice cream for breakfast at the Ice Cream Palace! They couldn't believe it. I was letting them have ice cream for breakfast! Hey, I wasn't about to go against this fine tradition. I think the fact that they were doing something that they never did before, made the ice cream taste even that much sweeter. To the kids' delight, after "breakfast," we met up with Grandma and Grandpa Shepard who flew in the day before so that they could join us on our Disney adventure. They had been there for us through so much, and now, it only seemed fitting that they were there to celebrate with us.

In the car, our excitement built even more as we passed various Mickey signs leading us to Disney. After parking, we took the free jitney to the tram that would take us right to the entrance. On the tram ride, I was able to get just glimpses of the famed Cinderella Castle and it was enough to get my heart beating just a little bit faster. With glee, I pointed and announced to the kids, "There's Cinderella's Castle!" You could see the awe and wonder in their expressions. The kids' enthusiasm was contagious and we couldn't get inside the park fast enough. This was the first time I had been to Disney World in years and I too got caught up in the thrill of it all. After handing in our tickets, we eagerly entered the park and found ourselves in a bustling square. As we rounded the circle, walking towards Main Street, U.S.A., there it was, Cinderella's Castle. Aaaahhhhhh. Even from a distance, it is an impressive and majestic sight. As we continued to walk, we got closer and closer to the castle, until we were right in front of it. Seeing it up close and personal, it is dramatic and grand. I don't care how old you are, when you see that castle in all it's wondrous glory, you are instantly transported to another world, another place and time. Grown-ups become kids again and kids believe that their best dreams can come true. It is indeed a Magic Kingdom.

There was so much to take in and of course, I took several thousand photos wanting to capture everything. After taking the proper time to admire the castle, we got right to it. Maddox and Danika couldn't wait to get on some rides. We rode on the classic merry-go-round, the iconic tea cup, and of course Dumbo, the Flying Elephant. Maddox loved riding The Barnstormer roller coaster and racing along the speedway. Danika delighted in Peter Pan's Flight and The Magic Carpets of Aladdin. We took an undersea journey with the Little Mermaid and sailed across A Small World. We met and got the autographs of almost all of our favorite Disney and fairy tale characters, including Mickey, Minnie, Tinker Bell, Princess Aurora, and Cinderella. From Fantasyland, to Frontierland, to Tomorrowland, we explored and enjoyed plenty of the park's attractions, too many to name.

One of the best parts of it all was that we never had to wait on any long lines. Not a one. As soon as the attendant saw the MAW badge that Brad wore and Maddy's GKTW pin, our family was immediately escorted to a separate "line" which brought us directly to the front. For those of you who have been to Disney, you are well aware of the massive lines and long waits at most of the attractions. To NOT have to wait on any long lines was a huge benefit. It allowed us to go on more rides and experience more of the park's activities because we didn't have to wait. This was the way it was at all of the theme parks, and also the way it was when we wanted to meet any of the characters. As soon as they recognized us as one of the Wish families, they brought us right to the front. MAW and GKTW really thought of everything to make this experience the best it could be, and it was. When the characters saw Maddy's pin, I noticed that they took special care to give him a little extra personal attention, either chatting it up, or goofing around with him just a little bit longer than the other kids. While they were of course attentive and playful with all the children, I must admit it was nice that they showed Maddox a little bit more love, probably understanding and knowing that this kid is as brave as they come. In fact, it made our whole family feel special in the very best way.

MAW generously provided tickets to all of the theme parks, one of which was Epcot. Rather than going to Epcot, which we felt was more for older kids and adults, we went to Magic Kingdom twice. On our second visit, I told Danika that we were "cordially" invited to have lunch with Cinderella at her castle! It was something special just for her. We talk a lot about how much Maddox has been through and rightfully so, but Danika also suffered and sacrificed so much when her brother was in treatment. She deserved this trip just as much as Maddox. Looking simply adorable dressed in her little Cinderella gown and fancy tiara, I watched my sweet baby girl's face light up when Cinderella greeted her at the castle. In fact, many of the princesses were in attendance at the Royal Table. Snow White, Princess Aurora, and Princess Jasmine each came to our table to say hello and take pictures with "Princess Danika," which was what they called her. It was fabulous. I watched Danika smile and curtsy with pride. She was having a "ball!" The happiness on her face filled my heart. Even I was honored to be in the presence of these beloved Disney characters. It was a royal treat! I loved sharing every moment of this magical experience with my daughter. Just me and my sweet girl. For so many reasons, it meant so much to me to enjoy this experience with just her. It may not make up for all those times I neglected her during Maddy's treatment, but it sure was a wonderful start. This "princess" lunch was a very special time for both of us, one that I hope she tells her daughter about when she is older. I know it is a memory I will always keep in a very special place in my heart.

While Danika and I enjoyed some Mommy and Daughter quality time, Brad and Maddox were experiencing their own thrills - roller coasters! The boys had their own adventures while the ladies were lunching. It was here that we, and Maddox, discovered his love for fast rides. Being the overprotective mom that I am, I often tried to dissuade him from some of those rides. Maddox was fearless wanting to experience all of them. Thankfully, there were restrictions on some of the rides not allowing younger children on them, otherwise the kid would have hopped right on all of them with a big smile on his face.

We all absolutely loved the extravaganza of the Disney Dreams Come True Parade in Magic Kingdom. Practically all of our favorite storybook characters came out for that one. There was Mickey, Minnie, Goofy, Donald, and Daisy. There was Cinderella's beautiful carriage float, complete with of course, her Fairy Godmother. Strutting down the street even Cinderella's stepmother and stepsisters got a roaring reception, although some of the little girls, including Danika, probably gave them looks of disapproval. The stepsisters kept bickering while stepmother stuck her nose up in disdain at the packed crowds. I must admit I was most amused by them as they were really playing the part. The actress in me loved it! The entire cast put on a great show. We watched excitedly as one character after another made an appearance on these vibrant and lively floats. There was a sparkly castle float with all the princesses and their princes waving to their throng of admirers. With big smiles on their faces, Maddox and Danika waved right back at them. There was Snow White with her dwarfs, an Alice in Wonderland float, and a myriad of dancers and singers to add to this already dynamic show. With the great music and all the pomp and circumstance, it was a fantastic spectacle of sight and sound.

MAW also got us tickets to Mickey's Very Merry Christmas Party, which took place in the evening. Because our trip was in November, the park was decorated with festive Christmas ornaments. As exhausted as we all were from the day's activities, we stayed into the night to attend this event - and it was well worth it. While Maddox was ready to party, Danika was somewhat cranky from being so tired. Keep in mind that we had already been in the park since the early morning, so for a little kid, it could definitely get a bit overwhelming. Well, Danika's tune quickly changed to giddiness once the evening's fanfare began. At the party, we were treated to an absolutely gorgeous light show on the castle and an electrifying fire works display. To all of our wonder and delight, we even saw Tinker Bell take flight as the castle and night sky glowed with colorful splendor. This was the first time the kids had ever seen a fire works show. It was wonderful to experience it with them and to see it through their eyes. Sitting there with complimentary hot chocolate and cookies, they ooohed, and wowed, and clapped joyously with the rest of us.

The whole week was a whirlwind of rides, shows, activities, and events. MAW spared no expense. Magic Kingdom, Hollywood Studios, Animal Kingdom, SeaWorld - we did it all! Just like Magic Kingdom, we never had to wait on any long lines at any of these other parks. As soon as a park's attendant saw the badge and the pin, our family was escorted to a sort of VIP separate line without delay. We were so thankful for that. It certainly made our experiences so much more pleasurable. At the various theme parks, we marveled at the kooky world of Dr. Seuss, we went on a wild safari, and we observed exotic sea creatures. At Hollywood Studios, Brad and I even got to visit Hogwarts! Being huge fans of the books, I have to admit that it was pretty cool. There really was something for all of us.

Throughout our week long vacation, we would spend our days in the parks, and at night, we enjoyed the special events and parties at the Village. Every day was packed with activities and adventures galore. At the Village, the kids got to swim, go on horse back rides, go to the Ice Cream Palace every day, and play in a life-size board game of Candy Land. One night, Maddox and Danika even had the unique pleasure of getting tucked in bed by Mayor Clayton. He tucked them in like a "burrito," as he called it, tucking the sheets in all around them, from their tippy toes to their shoulders, as they laughed and giggled. Even now, every once in a while, the kids would ask to get tucked in "burrito" style.

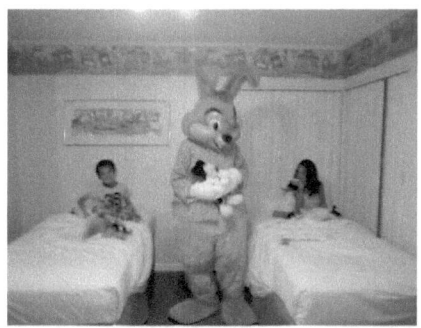

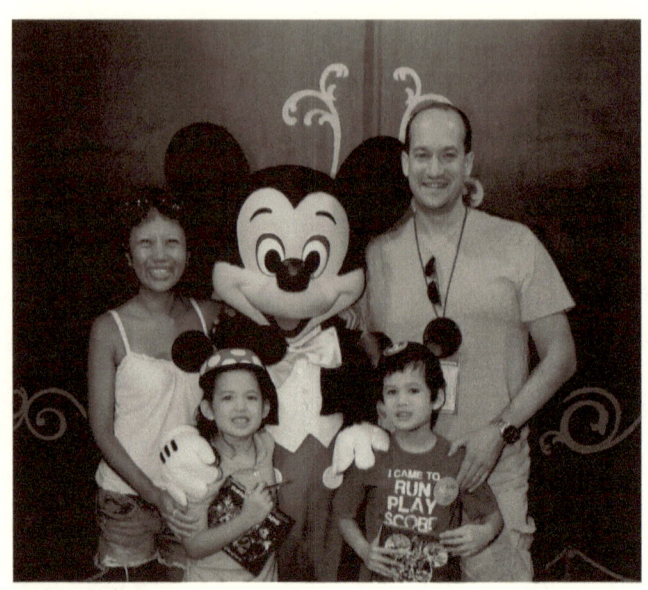

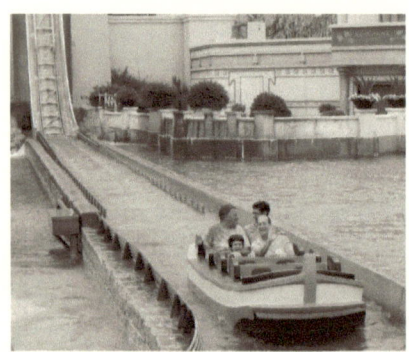

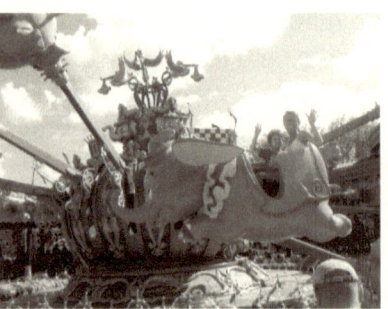

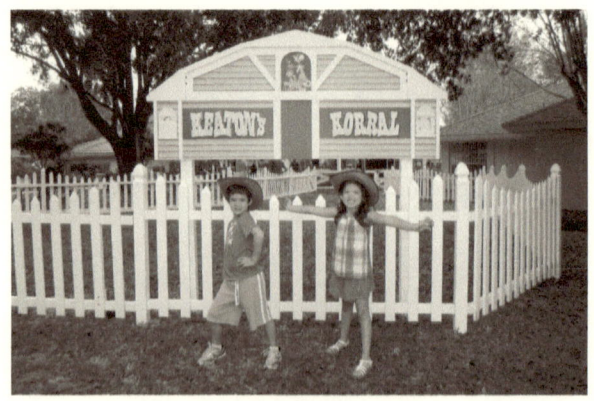

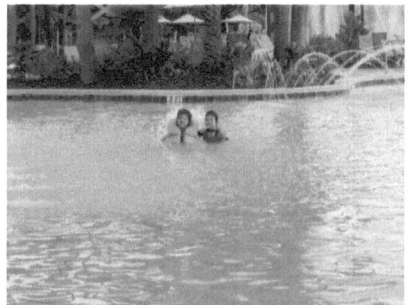
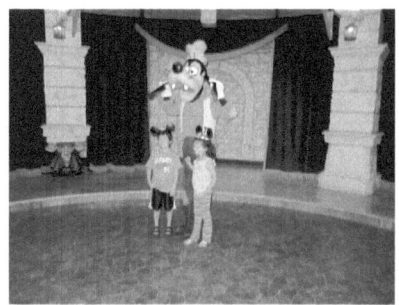

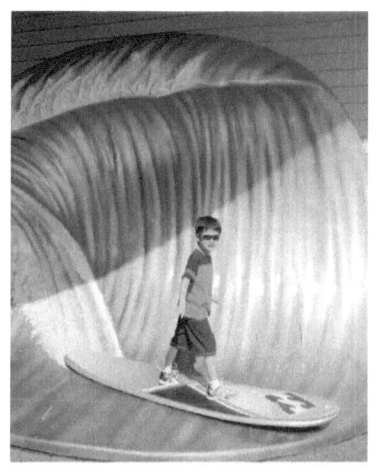
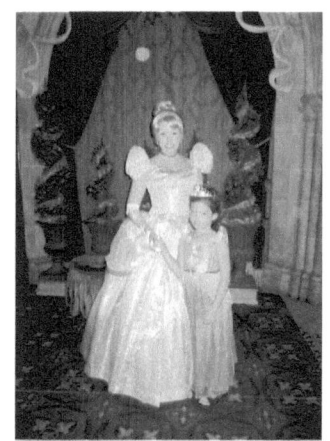

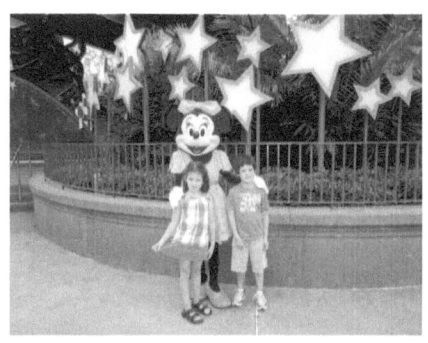
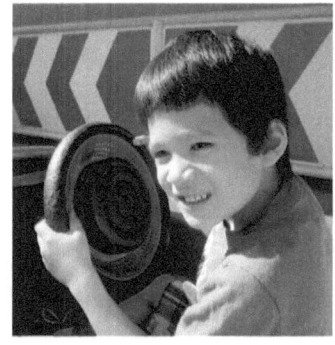

Chapter Eighty-Six

Our Disney week went by all too quickly, but before we left, we had the honor of including a star for Maddox in the Village's Castle of Miracles. This Castle of Miracles is unlike any other castle you have ever seen because it sparkles with the brilliance of the stars of all the Wish children that have stayed at the Village. It is a sight to behold with reverence. Maddox wrote his name on a bright golden star and it was placed among all the others, illuminating the walls and ceilings of this Castle.

When you go through what we went through when Maddox was in treatment, it was easy to think that we were the only ones. There were many days when it felt like it was only happening to our family. Standing there surrounded by literally hundreds, more like thousands of stars, I was reminded that it wasn't just us, that in fact, many, many families have suffered through the heartache and pain of taking care of a child with a life-threatening illness. We were not alone. The sight of it all can take your breath away. Each star represented a Wish child. Each shining star stood for the bravery and courage of so many, too many children. To grasp the number of stars inside this Castle was overwhelming. It can leave you feeling heartbroken and sad, but just for a moment, because then you realize how much happiness the Village brings to all of these children and their families. Each star also represented a Wish come true. For every star, there is a smiling face that got to experience the wonder and joy of the Village. That's what this place is - JOY!

On the day they showed us where Maddox's star was placed, I got very emotional. I love him so much. This special moment signified just how far he's come. This kid has been through a heck of a lot, but when you look at him, what you see is a happy, outgoing, kind, sweet, and good natured young boy. As I stood there looking at Maddox, looking at his bright star, I felt enormous pride. That's *my* son and he is *amazing*.

We as a family have endured so much and we survived it. I gazed at the thousands of glittering stars and took it all in with awe and respect for every fearless kid whose star was so lovingly placed on the walls and ceilings of this sacred Castle. For the fierce battles they have had to fight, they are all our heroes. With sincere admiration, I honored all of these children, including my own brave son. Maddox is a Survivor. He is an inspiration.

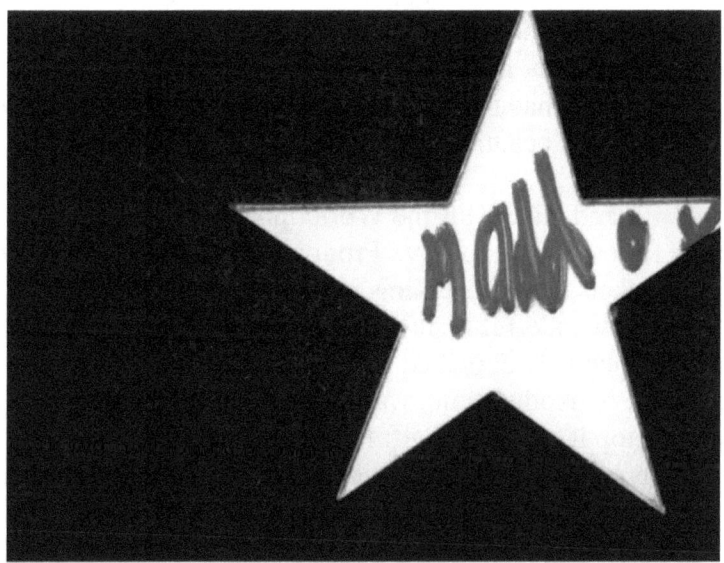

Chapter Eighty-Seven

I could write about and list all of the memorable moments and fantastic, amazing experiences we had at Disney and the Village, but there are way too many. This was the first *real* family vacation we've had in over three years. Brad and I were beyond grateful to finally be able to do this for our kids, for all of us. To go on vacations again is a simple luxury that we will never take for granted. Considering how long it has been, we were ecstatic to go on any trip, but this Disney vacation was truly a most *spectacular* one. The joy on Maddox's and Danika's faces every day, with each and every new delight, meant everything to us. After all the sacrifices they have had to make, to watch both of my children so happy was the most beautiful gift of all.

Make-A-Wish and Give Kids the World made this a magical experience for our whole family. From all of the complimentary theme park tickets to all the dining, especially the Ice Cream Palace, and the wonderful nightly parties in the Village, every aspect from when we got picked up by a stretch limo, to when we returned home in another limo, was thought of with so much love and care. To top it all off, the gift fairy came every day to the happy squeals of Maddox and Danika! Our family was incredibly moved with love by the thoughtfulness and generosity with which our trip was planned. MAW and GKTW thought of every single detail so that the only thing we had to do was simply enjoy it all.

We are so thankful to the Make-A-Wish foundation for the priceless gift of creating new and happier memories for our family. It was an amazing celebration for all of us. This vacation was truly a wonderful wish come true, one that we will forever treasure and never forget.

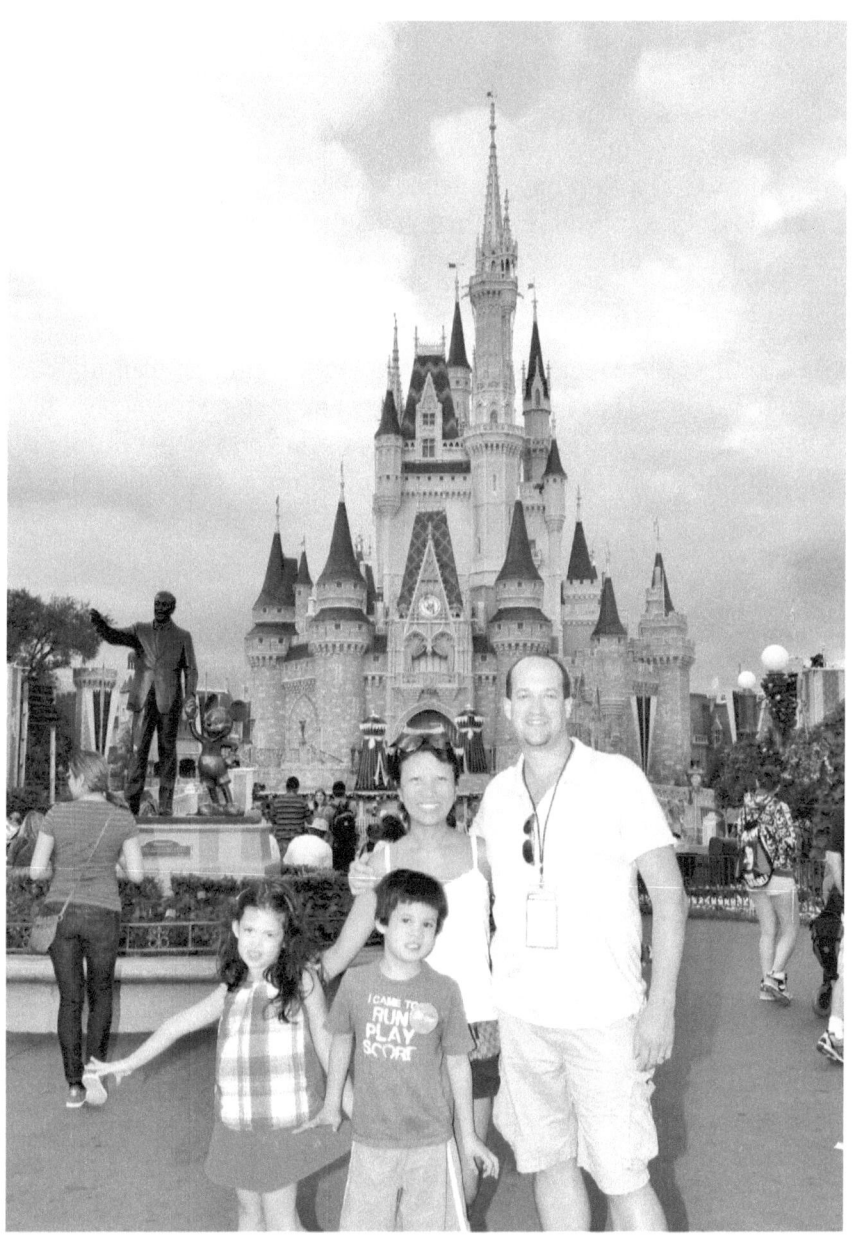

A Truly Magic Kingdom.

Chapter Eighty-Eight

It is May 2014.

So far, it has been almost two years since I began writing this book. I probably would have finished it sooner had I not been so afraid to look back on some of the events that shaped our lives. To look back was to relive all of those moments, many of them painful and heartbreaking. Once I started, I knew all of those memories that I had so carefully tucked away would rise to the surface with a vengeance. I wasn't sure that I could, or even wanted to go there, but I felt it was important to share our story. If this book somehow helps just one family or one person get through a difficult time, then I know that I did something good.

Chapter Eighty-Nine

Fallout

It is often said that it is after treatment that the enormity of what we went through really hits us. That is when we allow ourselves to truly take in the experiences of the past and feel all the emotions that we've bottled up for so long. More significantly, it is also when the dust settles, that the aftereffects of everything we've been through begin to reveal themselves.

I don't think it's possible to go through what we went through and come out unscathed. We are a product of our experiences and I fully admit that my past experiences have left me damaged. I don't think anyone, not even my husband, will ever truly understand just how much so. One of the toughest things for me is that I carry around this fear. Some days I feel like I am always afraid. This is the "baggage" that I talked about earlier. I know I said that I am doing my best to overcome these fears, and I am, but sometimes, old habits are hard to break. This crazy fear takes such control over me that oftentimes it holds me back from being the person that I want to be, the person my husband fell in love with. That girl was so easy-going, didn't read too much into things, and was not so quick to take everything said or done so seriously. She was outgoing and pretty much an open book. I miss her, almost as much as I'm sure Brad misses her. Don't get me wrong, I haven't completely lost all of those fine attributes. I know that I still have them in me, and I'd like to think that for the most part, I am still a fun-loving person, but there's no denying that my experiences have made me much more guarded, cautious, and certainly more private.

Most people would think that these issues I've developed are understandable considering everything that I've been through. A while back when I talked to a social worker, she likened what I was going through to PTSD, Post Traumatic Stress Disorder. She said it was very normal to experience fears and anxieties after going through not just my son's health scare, but also my own. Both events have certainly had its traumatic effects on me. For example, when I or anyone in my family gets any weird symptom, for a brief moment, my mind immediately goes to a scary place. It doesn't help that I've always had an overactive imagination. In those moments, I wish the rational part of me would just be calm and believe that it's nothing serious. Our history makes this so damn difficult. Right before Maddy was diagnosed, we took him to the pediatrician so many times concerned about the various odd symptoms he was having. They told us that it's perfectly normal for toddlers to often catch viruses and get over it. Each and every time they reassured us that it was "nothing." Well, as we all know, it was not "nothing." It was very much something. It was freakin' cancer! It has been almost a couple of years now since Maddy finished his treatment, but as I've said, every once in a while I still find myself dwelling on those earlier days when he was diagnosed. I really wish I knew how to get over it and move on. Brad seems to have done it. Why can't I??? One time, when Maddy got a fever after he was done with treatment, my first instinct was to call Dr. Gary to find out what we should do. For the years when Maddy was getting chemo, whenever he got a fever, that was the protocol - call the clinic. Now that Maddy was done, we didn't have to do that anymore. Dr. Gary simply replied, "Treat him like you would treat any other normal kid." It was the most glorious thing I had ever heard.

While Maddy has made a wonderful transition back to normalcy, it is taking me a bit longer to find my way there. I'm very aware that I've taken being an overprotective mom to another level, but it's because I had to. While Maddy was in treatment, we had to follow so many precautions. Eventually, it simply became a part of our day to day routine. I didn't know how to be anything else but protective. For months after Maddy finished his treatment, I still Purelled him and Danika more than was probably necessary. It was what I did for so long that it was kind of like a knee-jerk reaction. I have since gotten that under control. I have definitely given both my kids more freedom to get dirty just like any other kid, but I know that I still have a long way to go in terms of loosening up. It's almost as if I have to learn to be "normal" again. I have to change the way I think and react, like a cold in most cases, is just that, a common cold. I guess for me, settling into this thing we call "normalcy" is going to take some time.

Chapter Ninety

The experiences of the past have obviously left me with some emotional scars that may take a little longer to heal than others. There was a day Brad happened to mention that one of our friends posted on Facebook that she was pregnant. They have two beautiful children and were now expecting twins. My first reaction was not to feel happy for them, but instead, was to feel sad for me. I hated that I reacted that way. As much as I am ashamed to admit it, that was my gut, honest reaction. I felt like a horrible person and an even more horrible friend. Of course I wanted to be happy for them, but in the moment, I was too consumed with pangs of jealousy. I was diagnosed with breast cancer just as Brad and I were trying for a third child. Following that devastating diagnosis, our attempts to have another baby were suddenly and quickly derailed because I had to get chemo.

As awful as it sounds, hearing the news of our friend's pregnancy put me in a funk. I was sad because Brad and I couldn't have another baby. That thought led up to thoughts of why we couldn't - because I got breast cancer, which then led to thoughts of when Maddy and I were in treatment. Deeper and deeper I went. All of these painful thoughts collided together leaving me heartbroken and sad that our family has been through so much.

That night, in between tears, I confided in Brad. I told him how awful I felt that I made what was wonderful news for our friends, somehow all about me and my issues. There is a place of sadness in my heart whenever I think about when Maddy and I were treatment and what we endured as a family. That is a part of our lives that will always bring back unwanted memories and emotions. I told Brad that I think about our friends and the other people in our lives and how lucky they are that they have not known such sadness or pain. While I don't know all the details of their lives behind closed doors, on the surface, it just seemed like their happiness has not been tainted the way ours was tainted. Of course, I would never ever want anyone to go through anything like what we went through, but I couldn't help but agonize and wonder, "Why did it happen to us???" I know that train of thought is pointless, but sometimes, it is just too easy to go there.

I asked Brad if he ever gets sad when he thinks about everything we have experienced. He replied that of course he did, but he is more thankful that we got through it and that our family is doing well. He focuses on that. My head knows that he is right, but my heart still hurts whenever I reflect back on some of those difficult days. It has always amazed me how Brad or men in general can just easily brush things aside and not dwell in the past. It is an enviable skill. I know for me and perhaps other women, we have a tendency to just "live there" sometimes. As much distance as I put between me and the events of the past, I know that when I choose to remember, I can bring myself back there in a heartbeat. All the hurt and heartaches that go with those memories would not be any less painful. Trust me, I don't often choose to go back there, but sometimes, in the quiet of the day, my mind just wanders into forbidden places. Some things are simply hard to forget. I also know that when I feel, I feel things very deeply. I'm sure you have figured out by now that I am a sensitive soul. It's just who I am. It's how I'm built. It's crazy how this simple, yet exciting news of our friend's pregnancy led to such a serious and emotional conversation. Brad was probably like, "Get over yourself, Geri and let me go to bed!" I wish it was that easy to just "get over it." For some time after Brad fell asleep, I found myself lost in too many thoughts. Man, I feel so messed up.

As I mentioned, I was prescribed tamoxifen after my treatment as a preventive measure against cancer. I could not get pregnant while I am on this drug because of the adverse effects it may have on a baby in utero. Before starting chemo, I had the option to consider freezing my eggs. At the time, Brad and I never seriously considered it. It was quite expensive and really, our primary focus was on getting me through chemo and getting me well. Initially I was told I'd be on tamoxifen for five years. As I mentioned, at a check-up, my doctor told me that studies have shown that being on tamoxifen for ten years is proving most effective in survival rates. So now I am on this drug for ten years! By the time I'd be ready to unfreeze those eggs, I'll be in my fifties! I know some women are okay with that and would be very capable of having a newborn in their fifties. Not me. I think I'd be too damn tired in my fifties to be changing diapers and doing round the clock feedings. It just wouldn't be fair for a baby to be raised by parents who may not have the stamina to keep up with the growing needs of an active baby, then toddler. That is just my opinion. I know there are others that would think otherwise and that's totally fine. Let's face it, for me, now in my forties, I don't have as much energy as I had when I was in my thirties. Yes, I still consider myself pretty physically fit and know I would have been able to care for a newborn, but there's no denying that age plays a factor in our overall endurance. In my fifties, I'm not so sure I'd have the same amount staying power to keep up with the needs of a baby. So all things considered, I did not freeze my eggs. By far what made that decision for Brad and me even easier are the two purest joys of our lives, and that's our beautiful children, Maddox and Danika. With every fiber of my being, I thank God every day for them. They are the greatest blessings of my life. Wanting another baby never ever took away from the love that I have for them. It's because Maddox and Danika bring such immense joy into our lives that the thought of having another baby would have added to that. Brad and I love our family so much. We just felt like we had so much love to give.

For several months, Brad and I flip-flopped on whether to try for another baby. When we finally did decide to have another go at it, breast cancer happened to me. We figured that was that. The decision was made for us. For the most part, I have made peace with this, it's just that when I hear about a friend's pregnancy or even when I see a pregnant woman on the street, I can't help but feel this longing. I'd think about how wonderful it would be to give Maddox and Danika a baby brother or sister. I'd think about holding he or she in my arms and taking in that sweet delicious scent that only a newborn baby has. I'd think about how extraordinary it would be to feel this life, this miracle growing inside of me one more time. Then, in that same moment, I'd realize that it wasn't meant to be. Breast cancer took that choice away from me and that's what hurts the most. So yeah, when I think about it, it makes me just a little bit sad. Let me be very clear, this absolutely does not mean that I am not grateful for my kids. Having a third child would have been amazing, but Brad and I already know, with all of our hearts, that we have so much to be thankful for in Maddox and Danika. In both of them, we have everything.

Chapter Ninety-One

I know that I've developed some "issues" that need to be resolved. As I heal emotionally, I continue to be a work in progress. Brad sometimes jokes around that I am a control freak and I can't really argue with him. I've also heard Brad's mom make on the side comments about me being OCD whenever she observed me cleaning up the kids toys so meticulously, or whenever I put something back in it's "right" place. She too would be just "joking" around but I knew that while they said it jokingly, it was what they really thought. A part of me would be hurt and annoyed whenever they made those remarks because it made me feel like there was something wrong with me. The other part of me felt ashamed because they weren't too far off the mark.

To be honest, I don't remember ever being that way when Brad and I first met or when we were dating. I remember being so carefree and laid back. Well, cancer can sure knock that right out of you. I probably had some of those control and OCD tendencies in my nature, but after everything we have been through, those tendencies became more magnified. There were moments that I wanted to confide in them the reasons for my behavior, but it never seemed to be the appropriate time. I guess in a way, this is my opportunity to explain to Brad and others why I feel such a need to be in charge of what seems like everything. It's because for the three and a half years that Maddy was in treatment, and during my own treatment, I felt like I had absolutely no control over anything. My son got cancer and then I got cancer! What the hell was happening?! There wasn't a damn thing I could have done to prevent it. It was one thing when it came to me, but when it came to my son, it tortured me that I wasn't able to protect him from this. It felt like our lives were so out of control. Helpless. Powerless. Those are some hardcore scary feelings. Because of that, I clung, and I mean clung, to anything that I could control. In order to maintain balance and my sanity, I found ways to compensate for the lack of control I had in our situation. For example, I not only became a control freak, I became a clean freak as well. I wasn't able to change the fact that my son and I were getting chemo at the same time, but I sure knew that I could clean the hell out of my kitchen. As preposterous as that sounds, it became one of my coping mechanisms. I was desperate to find control in something, in anything. For some strange reason, when everything around me felt out of control, I found a sense of stability in a well-kept kitchen. Cleaning. Organization. Order. That's how I learned to deal. Even after Maddy and I finished our treatments, I didn't know how to not be a control and neat freak. It's what I became. I'm finding it hard to release the "grip" because doing so would mean letting go, and that scares the hell out of me. I am very much aware of this behavior and strive every day to loosen up.

Chapter Ninety-Two

This need for control has manifested itself in other ways. This is
where things are going to start sounding bizarre, but stay with me.
It's an issue that I've been afraid to fully discuss. It's not the
easiest thing to explain. Maybe only others who have experienced
something similar can understand. There are many moments when
I feel like I am living life being so careful about what I say and
what I do - careful about so many details. The decisions that I
make are all rooted in this overwhelming need to keep my family
safe. That is what is really at the core of it all. In my mind, and
obviously based on our experiences, I know that I can't protect us
from everything, but that hasn't stopped me from trying. I became
very superstitious and in the process, developed some strange
phobias.

Truth be told, I know how I came to be this way. There was an
incident that occurred several months before Maddy was
diagnosed. Somehow, in my warped way of thinking, Maddy and
then me getting cancer, was the result of that incident. Trust me, it
is a thought that most people would describe as outlandish. No
one in their right mind would have made the association, but me
and my superbly crazy thoughts went there and created this absurd
connection between the events. It was not based on any reason or
logic, but instead it was based on fear. I am not ready to discuss
what that event was and I'm not sure I ever will be. I don't mean to
sound so mysterious, but I am genuinely scared to talk about it.
Perhaps only a "professional" can get me to talk. The fact that I
am even mentioning it now is kind of a small breakthrough for me.
All I can say is, it was that event that reinforced my superstitions
and phobias.

If you recall, I wrote about these issues before I was diagnosed
with breast cancer. I was letting irrational fears get the best of me.
After I was diagnosed, I thought I had rid myself of this behavior.
I thought I had learned my lesson that succumbing to irrational
fears was pointless and a waste of energy. When I was going to
learn that we can't control everything?! You'd think that after

knowing first hand, and being face to face with real fear - a.k.a. cancer - that I would have put an end to all of these foolish and abstract notions. Somehow, my phobias and fears have found a way to rear their ugly heads.

Once again, I thought that I could keep harm away. It got to the point where I would behave and do or not do something based on these superstitions thinking that I could prevent anything bad from happening. It's almost as if I became a slave to my phobias and superstitious beliefs. It is mentally exhausting. It is debilitating. It is frustrating. Yet, I continue to let them control me. Even now, I can't give specific examples of the things that I did or what my phobias are because I am too scared to write them down. People are going to think I'm crazy. Heck, I think I'm a bit coo coo crazy. I know that my overactive mind takes me to some strange places. It's just that after everything that my family and I have been through, I wanted to "earn" us as much good luck as I could get. In order to do that, I let superstitions influence many of my actions. I know this may sound ridiculous and not make sense to many people, but somehow it was another way that I learned to cope. Brad would wonder and be baffled sometimes about the way acted. That is why. It was how I thought I could somehow protect our family.

Believe me, I know all too well how "things" can just happen and how there are just things in this life that we can't control no matter how hard we try. Yet, a part of me still thought that somehow I could. I know that it is not okay to live life in fear of what may or may not happen. As the saying goes, "A life lived in fear is a life half lived." I know all that. But still, there are two sides of me that seem to constantly be at war. There is the strong side of me that lives each day appreciating every moment, not taking anything for granted. Thank holy goodness for that side. Then there is the weak side of me that makes decisions based on irrational thinking and phobias. I am ashamed that I often put more trust on superstition instead of putting more trust in my faith. That is the internal battle I struggle with. I especially hate it when my husband finds himself in the crossfire between those two competing sides of me, leaving him confused about my behavior. I was always too embarrassed to explain all of this to him. Brad is such a logical and reasonable person. He would never understand why I would allow superstitions and phobias to influence me so much. It's basically because I'm so damn scared!!! I don't want any more bad things to happen to us. It must be very frustrating for him whenever I did something kooky all in the name of protecting our family. The rational part of me - and there is one, thankfully - knows that there's no guarantee that all of these "things" that I do will keep us safe. Of course I know that these beliefs are not based on any reason and knowledge. But I am just so afraid of what might happen if I didn't do the things that I did. I got so used to being this way that it's hard for me to just let go of this nonsensical thinking and acting. At the same time, I feel like Brad should be more sensitive and understanding of the fact that I have very deep emotional scars that are still healing - some of which may never heal completely. How I'm dealing with them may not make any sense, but they became ways for me to cope. I suppose you can call these issues that I've developed, the "fallout" from everything we have been through. I may look like I have it all together, but in some ways, I'm kind of fucked up. That may be an overstatement, but sometimes, that's how I feel. Many people would probably agree after reading this chapter. Talk about taking PTSD to a whole other level.

Sure, I have those moments when I think, "Hell yeah, I beat cancer! Carpe Diem!," but underneath all that bravado, there is that underlying fear.

Some of you may be wondering why I included this odd chapter. I guess it's because it's a part of my story. I want people to know that after a traumatic experience, or in my case, a couple of traumatic experiences, not everybody bounces back so easily. Some people find productive ways to cope, while others, such as myself, find more unusual ways. The important thing to understand is that we are all just doing the best we can. Even long after treatment is done, some us still find ourselves picking up the pieces, doing our best to recover mentally and emotionally.

I know that I have to find a way to work through and resolve my crazy issues. Just admitting to all of this is a big deal for me. It is an important step taken towards facing my fears. Random things happen in this life. I have to trust that God and the guardian angels above are watching over us. My faith has gotten me through some tough times and ultimately, I know it is my faith that will save me. I just have to find the courage to let it.

Change can be terrifying, especially when certain behaviors have become so ingrained in you. It's kind of like going through withdrawal. I have to resist every urge to act on old detrimental impulses until they no longer have a hold on me. It will take some time and lots of willpower, but I know that in order to live a better and fuller life, it has to be done.

I can not, I *will not* be defined by my fears. I have to summon the courage to not be afraid anymore and live. Live without hesitation. Live without fear. Just, live. LIVE.

Chapter Ninety-Three

Reflections

Thinking back, there were moments when we were at the clinic or one of those St. Baldrick's events, that I would look at a family and know all too well their looks of weariness and despair. I wish I could tell them that they were not alone, that they will get through it. It was those moments that inspired me to keep writing.

We were at a St. Baldrick's party one day and there was a mother who shaved her head in honor of her son who was battling a life-threatening illness. She was in tears and all I wanted was to tell her that she was not alone in the fight. I wanted to tell her about us, about Maddox, about our journey. I was hesitant, but felt compelled to say something to her to ease her pain. Finally, I gathered up the nerve to approach her. I wanted to say so many things and let her know that as a mother, I understood everything she was going through, but in that moment, all I could do was go up to her and say, "You're amazing. It's not easy, but it does get easier." She seemed a bit taken aback. I think she just smiled politely and said thank you. Afterwards I felt a little foolish wondering whether that was the right thing to say. I remember thinking that if I just had my book, this book that I am writing now, I could have given that to her and simply said that I hoped my story would help her get through some tough times, and perhaps provide her with some strength, support, and comfort. While my grammar and use of punctuation and language may not be perfect, this book is written from the heart, and with the very best intentions. I'm sharing our story in the hopes that moms like her, and others going through difficult situations, will know that we are all stronger and capable of so much more than we ever thought we could be.

Chapter Ninety-Four

In March of 2013, our family was invited to speak at a St. Baldrick's event hosted by the company NetApp, a strong supporter of the St. Baldrick's Foundation. When we were first approached to share our story, I was a bit reluctant. I knew that Brad wasn't going to do the talking so it was up to me to be the voice for our family. I wasn't sure that I could get up in front of a crowd of strangers and basically pour my heart out to them, but at the same time, I knew that it was really important to raise awareness for childhood cancer. If we could play a small part in doing that, then it was our responsibility to do so. Many people raise money for St. Baldrick's and other charities like it, but don't really get a sense of what they're supporting and what they're fighting for until they witness first hand what childhood cancer does to a family. We would be the face of what that event was all about. We raise money for childhood cancer research so that one fine day, no more children and no more families have to go through what we went through. I knew going up there and telling our story would be tough, but I also knew that it would make this cause very real and very personal for everyone there.

As I prepared my speech, I thought, "How in the world was I going to consolidate three and a half years in just five minutes???" Well somehow I did it, and in the process, similar to writing this book, it was like the events of the past replayed in my mind filling me with so many emotions. Writing this speech was one thing, but reading it out loud was not going to be easy. The first time I read it aloud in my living room, I was a hot mess, barely able to get to the second paragraph before I was balling uncontrollably. I certainly did not want embarrass myself and do that in front of all those people! I figured, let me practice several times so by the time I do it for real, I will be composed.

The night of the party, I was so nervous. We arrived and were the guests of honor. I was told that we would be ushered to the side of the stage when it was time for me to speak. It was held at some nightclub type place. They had a nice buffet and music. I love a good buffet, but I was so anxious waiting, I could hardly enjoy any of it. Maddox and Danika enjoyed themselves on the dance floor, frolicking and dancing around, while Brad and I stood by some nearby banquettes watching them. At one point I think I said to Brad, "Do you want to do it?" to which he replied, "This is your thing, Geri," referring to my early acting days. You'd think with a background in acting that speaking in front of an audience would be a piece of cake, but as an actress, your job is to be somebody else. This, on the other hand, was all me. There was no hiding behind a role or a character to play. This was as real as it gets.

There were already a lot of people there and it was loud. The first thing that went through my mind was whether anyone would even listen to me. I wondered whether I would be standing there on this stage feeling foolish as everyone else just enjoyed the party eating, drinking, and talking. Whatever. I quickly brushed those thoughts aside. We were there for an amazing cause and if only hand full of people paid attention to me, then so be it.

Soon, the music stopped and the master of ceremonies got up to the stage and welcomed everyone to the event. As he spoke about his company and its participation in the head shaving fundraiser, our family was brought closer to the stage. A moment later, he was introducing us, "Without further ado, we'd like to bring the Shepard family up." Oh my gosh, this is it. Will people listen? Will anybody care? While my right hand held, more like gripped the microphone firmly, my left hand that was holding my speech, trembled with anticipation. I took a deep breath and with Brad, Maddox, and Danika standing beside me, I began our story.

As the words came out, the crowd began to gradually hush until the only noise I heard was the sound of my voice. It was so quiet. Every once in a while, when I dared to look up from my speech, all I saw was everyone's attention on me. At one point, I lost my spot reading the speech and I had to pause for a moment. I almost started to panic, but then I felt Brad's hand rub my back in reassurance, and I found my way again. Not surprisingly, I did not make it half way through the speech before my voice broke and tears welled up in my eyes as I told all of these people what we went through when we found out that our little boy had cancer. Although I was able to I hold my tears at bay, refusing to let them fall, my voice was unsteady and my emotions were very, very raw. Keep it together, girl You got this. Glancing around I could tell that many others, some with tears in their eyes, were getting caught up in our story too. The emotions seemed to have filled the room as all of these people were hearing first hand what childhood cancer does to a family and how it robs these children of so much of their precious childhood.

I continued on with our story saying, "Cancer is cruel regardless of your age, but for a child, it is devastating. It robs these kids of a part of their childhood. When they should be going to playgrounds, playing sports, and having play dates, these kids are getting chemo. It is heartbreaking. We know this because we lived it. We are thankful today because we survived it!"

It was at those words that my face lit up and my voice regained its strength. With joy and gratitude in my heart, I announced that Maddox finished his treatment in August of 2012!

Before wrapping up my speech, I thanked all of the head shaving participants and NetApp for supporting such an amazing organization. More importantly, I couldn't finish without introducing the little man of the hour. With pride, I put my arm around my son and said, "This is Maddox. He is a Survivor." In an instant, the room ROARED with thunderous applause to honor and acknowledge my brave boy. I looked out at the crowd and practically everyone was on their feet clapping wildly for Maddy. Wow! The response was Powerful. It took me a bit by surprise. I must admit it was kind of exhilarating. I was overcome with emotion and pride. Maddy just stood there smiling, not truly comprehending that the enthusiastic applause was all for him. He certainly deserved it. What a truly incredible and memorable moment for our whole family.

I gave the microphone back to the host who then introduced Maddy to Justin Tuck, defensive end for the NY Giants. At these events, the sponsors often get celebrities and athletes to participate in the head shaving to help raise money and awareness for the cause. Maddox had no clue who the big guy was, but gladly shook his hand and accepted the presents, which included an autographed football, that this well-known athlete was handing him.

While Danika also got some nice gifts, I remember her later making a comment saying something like, "Why does Maddy get all the attention?" It wasn't those exact words, but it held that same meaning. Immediately, it brought back all of those feelings of guilt that I had about neglecting my daughter while Maddy was in treatment. My heart sank at the thought that Danika was once again feeling like she was taking a back seat to her big brother. The only thing I could think of to comfort her in that moment was to tell her that she had gotten presents too. I knew it was a lame response. She may be young, but Danika has always been a very perceptive child. She was right. Despite my best efforts to appease her, she knew that her brother was the center of attention that night. How could I explain to her why her brother was the focus? It wasn't because he is loved more, or is smarter, or is more talented than her. It is because her big brother had cancer. No parent in the world would ever want that attention for their child. We as sure as hell didn't. How I wished to God that my little boy didn't have to fight that battle, but he did. Explaining that to Danika would be a conversation we'd have another time, perhaps it would be soon, or perhaps it would be when she's a bit older so that she could really understand why her brother got so much recognition. Maddox is a cancer Survivor and for all that he endured and conquered, our little boy deserved that praise. All I could do is hope and pray that Danika always knows that she is loved as equally and as fiercely as her brother. I promised myself that I would always make sure that she knew that.

As the music pumped back on, the mood was festive and bright as both of our kids took pictures with some famous football players. Immediately after we got off the stage, our family was greeted with lots of hugs and handshakes, and with Maddy getting lots of high fives. Danika forgot her earlier concerns giggling with delight as her daddy hoisted her up and carried her on his shoulders. Thankfully, it was as simple as that to make her happy again. We weaved our way through the crowd as various people approached us and said, "Your family is amazing" and "God bless you" and "That was an incredible speech." Others said, "You're an amazing mom" and "You guys are incredible" and "Thank you for sharing your story." All around us the show of support was overwhelming and filled us with gratitude and love. In a cab on the way home, I felt very proud. We did good.

Chapter Ninety-Five

Sometime that night, I can't remember whether it was at the party or when we got home, Maddy said to us, "That story was about me!" He looked at us so happy with himself, and he said it with such wonder and amazement in his face. He was six years old at the time and old enough to understand most of what I was saying. He may not have picked up on every detail, but he certainly got the gist that the speech was about him. When I was standing there speaking in front of all those people, it never dawned on me that the most important person in the audience that night, would be my son. For a second, I did not quite know how to respond to my son's profound revelation. I realized that was the very first time Maddy had ever heard his story. I could only imagine what he must have been thinking listening to all the details of what he and our family experienced. Hearing the word "cancer," he may not have fully understood what it was, how can any child comprehend it? Adults can't even comprehend it. It is an awful monster. All Maddy knew was that he had to take this "medicine" for a long time. While he was in treatment, Maddy probably realized at some point that he was different from his friends, but now after listening to his story, he may have understood why.

Looking at him with so much love I simply said, "Yes Maddy, that story was about you." I told him about how brave he was with taking all the "medicine," and how thankful we all were that he is done with all of that. He beamed with pride and said, "That was a celebration for me!" With a big smile, I agreed and hugged him close. Indeed it was, Maddy. After a long journey, it was a very meaningful and moving moment to be able to stand there as a family, and say that we made it through and survived it! That night was a celebration for all of us. Later that evening, I thought it was perhaps time for Brad and I to sit down with our children and talk to them about those three and a half years that changed all of our lives.

Since the night of the party, Maddy was so curious, asking lots of questions about how he got sick and what happened to him. I promised him that soon we would all sit down together as a family and talk about it. He was very impatient and adamant, constantly asking every day, "Can you tell me my story now? Can I hear it now?" I didn't want to do it in between activities or school work. I wanted to choose a moment when there would be no distractions. When that day came, Brad and I didn't really prepare what we were going to say. Goodness knows that we knew the story all too well. It was an important conversation and all we wanted was to talk to our children about it, as simply and as honestly, as we could. Sitting on the couch with Maddox and Danika in between us, Brad and I began.

"Maddy, when you were two years old, we found out you were sick. You had yuckies in your body and the doctors had to give you medicine called chemo to make the yuckies go away."

"Did I have cancer?"

"Yes, Maddy, you had cancer, but you are all better. We got rid of all the yuckies."

We had first heard this term "yuckies" to describe pediatric cancer through another family whose daughter is also a cancer survivor. This family was involved in a fundraising event which we participated in called, Kids Walk for Kids with Cancer. The name of their team was, "Bye Bye Yuckies." When I heard it, I thought that it was a very clever way to describe cancer in such a way that little children can understand it, without it being scary. So when it was time to talk to Maddy about what happened to him, we used that term.

After responding to Maddy's question, I pointed to his chest and said, "Remember you had that port. That's where they gave you the medicine." Maddy looked down at his chest and I watched him as his hand lingered on the place where the port used to be. I said, "You were very brave getting all those pinches."

Then I made sure to look at Danika as I said, "Danika was a very good sister to you, Maddox. She was your only friend when we had to keep you home, and she helped Mommy and Daddy take really good care of you. We are so proud of you, Danika." At hearing this, Danika simply smiled shyly, impressed with herself.

Maddy continued, "So the party where Daddy shaves his head is a celebration for me not having cancer."

"Yes, it sure is. It is a party for you and for all the other brave children."

"So I go to the clinic to make sure there is no more cancer."

Inside, I said a heartfelt prayer to God for Maddy's continued good health, and then I looked at my son and said, "That's right, Maddy. At the clinic you have those check-ups to make sure there is no cancer."

Throughout the conversation, Brad and I covered various topics. Danika just sat quietly listening. I hoped that this talk would give her a better understanding of why her brother sometimes got more attention. Maddy was more fascinated. We talked about his days at the hospital and how we were all so happy when we brought him home. We talked about how the chemo made his hair fall out, just like Mommy when Mommy had to take the "medicine." I told him about how he hated taking the chemo at first, but then later was the one reminding me when to give it to him. We talked about the people that helped to get him well, like Dr. Del Toro and Dr. Gary. We talked about the great day when he finished his treatment. We talked about a lot of things, and by the end of the conversation, Maddy seemed pretty pleased with himself. We knew the kids were too young to go into all of the specific details of those three and a half years. Overall, I think Brad and I did a good job keeping the story simple, but with enough information to satisfy the kids' interest. When we were done, we told Maddox and Danika how very much we love them, and then we all had a big family hug. Some day when they are older, they can read this book and know exactly what our family went through and how we all survived it.

Chapter Ninety-Six

Transformations

Since finishing his treatment, Maddox's physical strength has improved by leaps and bounds. I remember one day, just one or two weeks after he finished chemo, I saw a remarkable improvement in his endurance. I first noticed it on those monkey bars in the playground. Maddy could never get through all of the rings, he always seemed to lose steam somewhere in the middle. All of sudden, there he was, zipping through it, with what appeared to be very little effort. With the chemo out of Maddy's system, Maddy's body was regaining its strength. His energy was also much improved. It was as if his body was learning to catch up with what it knew it was capable of. When he runs, there is so much power and force behind it, not to mention speed. Many days, when we walk home from school or some other place, Maddox likes to run as he gets closer to our building. In awe, I'd watch him and just like that movie, *Forest Gump*, I'd feel like shouting, "Run, Maddox, run!" With the wind blowing his hair back and the power in his running stride, I'd watch him and feel just incredibly thankful. There is nothing holding him back and I love that. I really, really love that.

His strength wasn't the only thing that improved - so did his appetite. I remember all too well when I was on chemo how almost everything tasted just awful. I could barely eat a thing. I was on chemo for three months. Maddy was on chemo for practically three and a half years. Needless to say, it must have really done a number on his taste buds. After finishing treatment, Maddy started trying all sorts of foods - and loving it! He has become more adventurous, willing to try all different kinds of cuisines. Before, he just ate his basics, his go to meals that he always liked, never really wanting to try anything new. Now, he pretty much eats everything I put in front of him at the table, including an assortment of vegetables. It's awesome! Since finishing his treatment, Maddy has gone through a wonderful transformation.

As we began to have more normalcy in our lives, Danika also blossomed. She is no longer that fearful and shy little girl. Her personality has really shined. She is smart, funny, goofy, and the most affectionate, and thoughtful little girl. Since starting school, Danika has found her confidence, becoming more social and at ease with herself and with others. This is the outgoing daughter that we knew was always there.

One of the other things that we noticed about Danika is that she has an incredible memory. Gosh, there are so many things that I wish she would forget, but every once in a while she'll make these comments that make me realize just how much she remembers from the past. One time, when we were talking about when Maddy was in the hospital, Danika chimed in and said something like, "Oh, I remember that. That was when Mommy and Daddy left and I had to stay home." Ouch. Those words cut like a knife. It hurt me to think that she still carries those memories with her.

On another occasion, she woke up crying from a bad dream. It seemed to have really shaken her up. When I asked her to tell me what it was about, she refused and with tears streaming down her cheeks, she just said that she was scared. I told her not to be afraid and that it was just a bad dream, that it wasn't real. I held her close as she slowly calmed down. After several tries to get her to open up, she finally confided in me that she dreamt that me and her daddy "went away." My heart fell and I immediately flashed back to when we had to leave Danika at home with her grandma so that Brad and I could take care of Maddy at the hospital. I can only surmise that that was the source of her fears, and that these fears had somehow manifested itself her dreams. How I wished I could take all those painful memories away from her. I looked at my daughter's sweet and anguished face and hugged her even closer. I told her how much Mommy and Daddy love her, that we would never leave her, and that we are always there for her.

Since then, Danika hasn't had any more dreams like that. Thank goodness. I'd like to think that it's because we have earned her trust once again, and her sense of security in our family has been restored. I hope that in time, thoughts of those days will continue to fade until they are just a faint and very distant memory for her.

Another time, Danika showed off her keen sense of memory once again. We were all sitting at the table having dinner when Maddy said, "Mommy, your hair is getting so long. Are you going to cut it like last time?" I replied back, "Mommy didn't cut her hair." Before I had a chance to explain, Danika quickly said to her brother, "Remember, Mommy had to take that special medicine that made her hair short." Of course she was referring to when I was on chemo. I sat there in utter amazement. This girl remembers everything!

These days when Danika comments about something that she or we as a family experienced in the past, she says it very matter-of-factly. She doesn't seem hurt or upset when she makes these remarks. This leads me to think and to hope that somehow she has found a way to make peace with it. I know that Danika probably has some scars from the past. We all do. As time goes on and as we continue to replace old memories with new and happier ones, I have to believe that those scars will heal for all of us.

As for me and Brad, we are in a much better place. In February of 2014, Brad had gotten a message from someone regarding The Leukemia and Lymphoma Society's, "Man and Woman of the Year" campaign. The rep wanted to find out whether we would be interested in participating in the fundraising event. Brad happened to copy me on the e-mail he sent to the rep. I was on a TV set doing some background work when I read it. These were his exact words, "*I actually think my wife would be a better candidate, as although we both went through a lot, she took much of the brunt in supporting Maddox.*" My eyes filled with tears because what he wrote truly warmed my heart. That simple statement meant so much to me.

Later we realized that the title may actually be awarded to the man and woman who earn the most funds. However, based on Brad's reply, he must have thought that it was awarded to those who were most deserving, and he thought that I was one of those people. I got emotional because this was the first time I ever witnessed Brad acknowledge that I took on most of the responsibility when it came to Maddy's care during his treatment. Before that, I must admit that I wasn't sure whether he really appreciated that. It always felt like it was just Brad's father who constantly gave me those props. I know it may seem like a selfish and trivial thing to want the credit, but I did. I needed that recognition from my husband. I saw his e-mail right around Valentine's Day. What Brad wrote in that message was the most romantic gift I could have ever gotten from him that day.

With regards to the hormone therapy, I have learned to manage the "moodiness" a bit better and that has made a difference in the way Brad and I communicate. I think we are both better listeners. I make more of an effort to think before I speak, and I especially do my best to step away when I am feeling particularly sensitive. Brad probably appreciates that the most. Even though we've said things that we'd rather not have said and have hurt each other along the way in this journey, at the foundation of it all is our deep love and respect for each other. Our marriage is not perfect. Sure, like many married couples, we sometimes drive each other crazy and find ourselves in very heated "discussions." We may not always agree, but what I know for sure is that we love each other very much. Our marriage has certainly taken some hits, but through it all, Brad and I have stayed true to each other and our family.

Chapter Ninety-Seven

The New Me

There is a lot of self-awareness and soul searching that happens after a going through a traumatic experience. Despite the issues I have to work through, I'd like to think that overall, I became a better version of myself. I know that may be hard to believe especially after revealing some of my interesting personality "flaws." Regardless of that, I can confidently say that there are some definite changes I have made within myself that I can be proud of.

It's interesting because I've noticed that some parts of me are much harder, and other parts of me have softened. Before, I was too polite, often sacrificing my own wants and needs for what others wanted. These days, I am more apt to speak my mind. In essence, I have become a more assertive person. My husband can attest to that. If I don't want to do something, I don't do it. If I feel a certain way about something, you better believe I will make it known.

This is especially true when it comes to looking out for my kids. As just an example, if my kids are near someone smoking, I will subtly move them and myself out of the way, or I would request that person to move. Some people may think that being exposed to the occasional second hand smoke is not such a big deal. Well it is to me, especially and particularly considering my and Maddy's history. There was a time when I would have just "politely" sat there cringing, too embarrassed to say something, while I allowed myself and my children to be subjected to second hand smoke. Not anymore. Now, I would find a way out or say something. This is easy when it comes to strangers. It can get a bit awkward however, when it comes to family or friends, whether it's that situation or something else. It's never my intention to be rude or disrespectful, especially to the people I care about, but when it comes to the good health and safety of my children, I will always, always put them first. If people get offended, then so be it. I would rather take the heat, then put myself or my children in an uncomfortable or unsafe situation. I guess in a way, I have shed that nicey, nicey part of me. I have to say that it is quite liberating not to have to be so "agreeable" all the time.

I have certainly become more outspoken when it comes to standing up for myself and my children. One afternoon, the kids were riding their scooters by the entrance to our apartment building - which many children do I might add. Maddy happened to zoom by an elderly woman. When we got to the lobby, I told him to slow down and to be careful and mindful of the people around him when he is scooting. He understood and said that he would. As we were heading to the elevator, that elderly woman that Maddy scooted by, stormed in front of me and started yelling, more like shrieking, at the kids and me, "You're children almost hit me with those scooters!" She caught the kids and me off guard. She went on and on and worked herself up into a frenzy. First of all, Danika was next to me, walking her scooter into the building, so I know she wasn't anywhere near this crabby broad and secondly, I had already spoken to Maddy about being more careful. It's not like Maddy was aiming for her or being malicious. Maddy never even touched her and she wasn't hurt. I guess it was enough to startle her, but that doesn't give her the right to scream at my children. I could tell that she was scaring them. So, I looked her straight in the face, and firmly said, "Please do not yell at my children. You need to calm yourself down. I already told my son to be careful and I will discipline my children about the scooters. Calm yourself. " I must have told this woman to calm down like five or six times. At one point, I heard Maddy, with such sincerity in his voice, say he was sorry to the lady. It was obvious that he felt awful about it. Here was my son, maturely taking responsibility for his actions, and she was too busy yelling to even notice. Perhaps if she took a moment to listen, she would have heard him apologize, and perhaps would have dialed it down several notches. About the fifth time I told her not to yell at the children, she finally paused and said, "Okay." She probably realized she was going too far. Eventually, she got in one elevator and we got into another, just so that we didn't have to listen to her rant anymore. My blood was boiling, but the whole time I refused to match her tone. I kept my cool. Honestly, she really could have approached that situation in a much more pleasant manner. I know I was proud of the way I handled it. The old me would have been embarrassed and mortified. The old me would have apologized and just kept everything she wanted to say inside. The new me on the other hand, was not that person anymore. The new me was not going to let anyone talk to me or my children that way. I was going to stand up for us.

When we got home, Danika said to me, "Mommy, when I heard that lady yelling, I wanted to cry." I told Danika and Maddox that the lady should not have yelled at them like that, and then with a smirk I said, "The only person that's allowed to yell at you - is me!" At that, they bust out laughing as they could tell that I was just fooling around. That lightened the mood and all was well. Amused, Maddy kept pointing out how many times I had to tell that woman to calm down. If I'm not mistaken, I think I saw a look of admiration in my kids' faces. I think they were proud of their mommy. I hope that I showed them that I will always have their backs.

Of all the positive changes I have gone through, the thing I'm most proud of is that I know am a much better mother. I know I talked about this earlier, but it is very true. Since finishing my treatment, I have become so much softer when it comes to my kids. I can honestly say that I truly enjoy Maddox and Danika each and every day. I have more patience and more understanding in the way that I mother them. I am human so like any other parent, I may lose my temper every once in a while, but never like the way that I did before. In the moments that I do lose my temper, after things calm down, I always, always take my kids aside and give them a huge hug and kiss and say, "I'm sorry that Mommy yelled, but even though I yelled, know that Mommy always loves you very much, no matter what." It is so important to me that my kids know how very much they are loved. These days, to avoid any lost tempers, I have learned to take a deep breath and allow a moment to myself so that I can approach the matter with a level head, and calmly diffuse and resolve whatever situation my kids may have gotten themselves into. It's a pretty good strategy. I have to say that I don't really have to use it very often because I have really good kids. I am not just saying that because I'm their mom. They really, really are good children. Of course like all kids, they misbehave on occasion, but for the most part, they are good listeners, very respectful, and well behaved. I am so very proud of the way Brad and I are raising them.

I really relish and love being a mother to these two amazing, funny, smart, thoughtful, talented, creative, and beautiful children. Some of the profound things they say and do are food for my soul. I hug and kiss Maddox and Danika several times a day, much more than I ever used to, and each time, it is always done with much passion. I close my eyes and take in every delicious second. I can't get enough of it, or them. I never take any of these precious moments for granted. There is so much emotion behind each show of affection because I am so thankful to be their Mama. The love I feel for them is deep as it is strong. They bring pure joy into my life.

Chapter Ninety-Eight

Time to Heal

After a particularly emotional day of writing, recalling the details of past events, I found myself feeling heavy and drained. It was often difficult to shake it off that sometimes when Brad came home from work, I would just be distant, carrying this sadness from remembering some of the things that we went through.

Even when I wasn't writing, there were times when the simplest, most random events would get me thinking back. It just happens. I go about my day, and something or someone would trigger an old memory. Every once in a while, something would remind me of the past and I would once again be haunted by those earlier days. Sometimes, when I drop the kids off or pick them up at school, I would look longingly at some of the very young siblings of Maddy's and Danika's friends. These toddlers are about one and two years old. With heaviness in my heart, I would just stare at them and think that that was how young and precious Maddox and Danika were when all that "mess" happened to our family. To this day, it is hard for me to look at a toddler without remembering what our lives were like when my kids were that young. Many of the memories I have of Maddy at that age involved being at the hospital, or giving him chemo, or being at the clinic. More heartwrenching than that, I have very few memories with Danika at that age because I spent most of my time caring for my son. When I look at pictures and videos of Danika when she was just one or two years old, looking as sweet as can be, with little curls in her hair, my heart just melts. She was just learning how to talk and the sound of her voice was so delicious. I lose myself in those memories. I look at photos of Danika back then and I just want to kiss her, hug her so very close, and hear her giggles. I'm desperate for it. I didn't get nearly enough of it before our lives were drastically changed.

I would feel so envious watching other mommies with their little ones, being so playful and untroubled, their joys untainted. I long for those days of playing with my kids as adorable little toddlers, with their cute baby faces and their cute baby voices, when our lives were simple and ordinary. I think about Maddox and Danika when they were that small and innocent and I just want more of it so, so much. I barely had a chance to enjoy and relish my kids at those tender, precious ages. Because of our unthinkable circumstances, it's almost as if I skipped through what I know would have been some of the most magical experiences with my little babies. You have no idea how much my heart aches to think about how we were all robbed of that special carefree time. Cancer took, ripped that away from us. We can't ever get that time back when we were just a "normal" family and it hurts. It still really, really hurts.

I guess that's why I sometimes found myself procrastinating when it came to writing this book. There were days when I just didn't want to go to some of those scary places or feel some of those awful, awful feelings again. Most people would just choose to forget, but I made a commitment to this project and to myself that I would get it done, regardless of the emotional toll that it would take on me. To do this book justice, I had to take a deep breath and gather the courage to travel back in time. I knew many of those memories were going to be painful, but the thing is, there were many wonderful memories as well. I just had to get through some pretty bad ones before I could get to the good stuff. Ultimately, it is the good stuff, the *great* stuff that made it all worth it.

Throughout our journey, as we faced some of the most difficult challenges, we also witnessed and experienced some beautiful things. We found beauty in a thoughtful gesture and a helping hand. We found beauty in the kindness of strangers. Most of all, we found beauty in the love and support of our family and friends. There was so much genuine caring, so much love, and so much generosity, not just from those we knew, but from so many wonderful people who we met along the way. It is inspiring.

Chapter Ninety-Nine

I know that I have been given a second chance at life. That may sound dramatic, but cancer is serious business. The fact that I survived it puts all sorts of things into perspective. I don't want to waste any moment of this precious life watching every move that I make and worrying about things that I can't control. Making peace with the past is not as easy as I thought it would be, but that's okay. Healing happens at its own pace. I know that I have some work to do to be the person that I want to be, the person that I can be proud of. As long as I continue to have faith and believe in myself, I know that I'll get there.

I am a cancer *Survivor*. That means something.

Even in our weakest moments, we are all capable of finding the courage and strength to rise above and overcome our challenges.

I've learned many things throughout this journey. Topping the list are a couple of important life lessons. I've learned that growing old in good health is a great gift, and that each new day on this beautiful earth is an opportunity to do better and be better.

I know that I must let the past stay in the past so that I can fully appreciate the here and now. It doesn't mean that I have to forget - because I won't. It simply means that I have to move forward and focus on all that is good in my life. I am so incredibly thankful each and *every* day to be a Mother to Maddox and Danika, to be here with my family, and to feel strength and good health in my body. Family. Good Health. Love. Those are the things that truly matter the most.

Chapter One Hundred

February 2015

It has taken me over two years to complete this project. As difficult and heartbreaking as it was to open myself up to some of those memories, I am glad that I did this. In these pages, I have bared my soul. In this book, my family and I now have a record, a memoir of the events that shaped and changed our lives, and made us who we are today. Some day, Maddox and Danika will read this book and when they do, they will know just how much our family has conquered. It is my hope that they will also know how special our family truly is, and that they are loved so very much.

I am most proud of my son. Maddox is an incredible little boy. I'm so grateful that Maddox has very little memory of all that he endured at such a young age and trust me, it was a lot. Despite the past, there is no hint of sadness or fear in him. Instead, Maddox is full of energy and enthusiasm. He is kind and gentle, so caring and affectionate. Most glorious of all, Maddox has a joy about him that is simply beautiful. It shines bright within him.

It was often Maddox's courage that got me through some tough days of my own. I would only have to look at my son to know that I too could be brave. He and I have been through a lot. In the face of our reality, we persevered. Together, we stayed strong and overcame the unimaginable. Maddy and I will always share a very special bond, beyond that of a mother and son. Two of a Kind. We are Survivors.

About the Author

Geri Payawal Shepard is married with two children. She graduated from the Fashion Institute of Technology with an Associate's Degree in Fashion Buying and Merchandising and a Bachelor's Degree in Marketing and Communications. Soon after graduating, she landed a job at WABC-TV's, *Live! with Regis and Kathie Lee.* It was there that Geri discovered her love for the performing arts. She later left the job to study and pursue a career in acting. She has worked in film, television, commercials, and print. This is Geri's second self-published book. The first book was a diary documenting her adventures in Los Angeles titled, *To Move or Not to Move to LA? One Actor's Journey to Find the Answer.* While she continues to audition and do occasional background work in film and television, Geri's primary focus and joy is being a stay-at-home mom, spending time with her family and raising her two beautiful children.

www.ingramcontent.com/pod-product-compliance
Lightning Source LLC
Chambersburg PA
CBHW030421290526
45786CB00001B/76